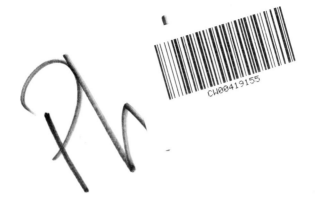

Little Dave's
Big Fitness Plan

I've heard all
about you!
keep it up!
Dave Cancau
X

For my daughters, Ella, Maya and Lula

Little Dave's
Big Fitness Plan

The hardest part is getting changed

Dave Concannon

First published in 2012 by
Concannon Press
28 Blandamour Way
Southmead
Bristol
BS10 6WE

A CIP catalogue record for this book is available from the British Library

ISBN 978–0–9574104–0–4

Brand and product names are trademarks or registered trademarks of their respective owners

Lovingly created by Infinite Authors

Printed and bound in Great Britain by TJ International Ltd, Padstow, Cornwall

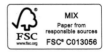

Contents

Starting at home 93

Introduction

I first started thinking about writing a book a few months after leaving the Royal Navy, in February 2005. By then I had been a qualified professional fitness instructor since January 1987. I had left to start my own fitness training business and on a good week would work with 25–30 clients. It was enjoyable and very satisfying, but there was a limit to who I could reach.

It surprised me that the people I met were making the same simple mistakes and struggling with the same challenges they had since I had become a fitness professional. I continued to work with more and more different clients. The techniques, coaching points and training programmes I used were based on simple formats for each individual but with subtle changes. They all worked and continue to work!

Information on exercise is easy to obtain, there is plenty of it – so much, in fact, that it can be difficult to know where to start, and easy to become confused and overwhelmed along the way. This book is intended to get you in the right frame of mind, to help you think positively and understand practically how to begin exercising and to continue forever.

In everyday life there are always challenges, setbacks, good and bad cycles. You deal with them because you know what is best for you, or because someone is there to help you. Exercise works in a similar way, but you can get stuck if you are badly informed or when things go a bit pear-shaped. That's when a small challenge becomes too big and you give up.

At heart, most people want to exercise – and everyone can. Sit down and think realistically about what you want to achieve. You'll soon realise that you *can* reach your goals. However, this book will not do the exercise for you! If you want to become fitter and healthier you'll have to make a sacrifice, pay the price and commit yourself to the cause. There's no such thing as something for nothing. But don't let that put you off, because everything I tell you in this book is simple, easy to understand and effective.

The big advantage is that I have had a go at plenty of different exercise programmes that I thought would be worthwhile. I've watched, read about and tried all sorts – programmes recommended by everyone from Arnold Schwarzenegger to David Beckham. Eventually I realised what might work for them won't work for me! So that should save you some time and sweat – you're already learning from my mistakes.

You *can* exercise for life. It's not just achievable – it's easy. You don't need luck, just a bit of mental preparation, a good routine and a sense of humour!

This book and why you should read it

I can bet you a rollover jackpot-winning lottery ticket there are no shortcuts to your health and fitness. Most of us take the long route and make it more difficult than it actually is. The exercise is the easy part.

I remember joining HMS *Boxer* in January 1988. At 23 years old I had been qualified as a Royal Navy Physical Training Instructor for one year. It was the first time I had been solely responsible for sport, recreation and fitness levels of the ship's crew of 220 Royal Navy, Royal Marines officers and men. We were due to sail to the Middle East for a seven-month deployment and patrol. I had high ambitions and hoped to encourage and motivate the whole crew to take part in exercise while we were away. Why not? There's always plenty of opportunity for exercise sessions while at sea. The flight deck of a ship, sea air and the sun coming up is a fabulous environment in which to exercise. Not only that, it is positive to exercise while working, sleeping and eating in a sometimes stressful environment. Of course, there isn't much hope of getting the bus home either.

I would like to tell you that I had everyone taking part in exercise, but from my experience the ship's crew was a reflection of today's society with regards to exercise. I classed about 15 per cent as the 'crazy gang'

– those who would exercise like their lives depended on it. At the other extreme was about 15 per cent who would rather swap their sports kit for a Pot Noodle (yes, you get those in the armed forces too), and would do everything they could to avoid exercise. There was about another 15 per cent of 'steady eddies', who were happy just cracking on with a little bit of exercise, pleased with what they were doing and generally weren't too fussed. No problems with that.

These first three groups all have one thing in common. They are all *consistent*. Consistently doing it, or consistently avoiding it!

So what about the other 55 per cent of the ship's crew? Here's the difference – these guys were *inconsistent*. They were generally a bit haphazard, going from nothing, straight to the crazy gang, and quickly back to the Pot Noodle brigade, or just starting and stopping as the whim took them.

If you're reading this book, you're probably a member of the 55 per cent gang. Maybe your exercise regime has been a bit haphazard in the past, or maybe you've had a few false starts. That's okay. All I need to do is get you to exercise *consistently* for the rest of your life. Don't be overwhelmed by the lifelong commitment, it's not what it seems.

There's nothing scientific about exercise in the armed forces, but it works. A young person joins up, you get hold of them, give them some physical objectives to aim for, and work towards it in a *consistent* way. Now, I know there's no such thing as 'one size fits all', and you may think that servicemen and women are different from you. But the basic principles I used on them work for people of all ages and abilities. You need to find a tempo and intensity that suits you, get your body moving in a safe and enjoyable way and do it *consistently*. That is exactly what I did with the 55 per cent gang. I gave them the routines and exercises outlined in the rest of this book.

The poor crew were stuck on a warship away from home and spent the majority of the seven months at sea. For me it was a perfect environment in which to work. I had the support of the captain who was keen to keep his men fighting fit, so he was the first one I harassed (tactfully) to exercise, and then worked my way down. There's no hiding place at sea, and I followed, pestered, sold, suggested, motivated, dragged and drove every member I could to exercise. I even suggested that the ship's padre should attend flight-deck circuits, and he suggested I attend church. So he did, and I did. That was the hard part – the rest was easy. Once they were exercising *consistently* they didn't want to stop, they couldn't get enough of it. It will be the same for you. The routines work, they are simple, varied and effective, and are easily adapted to suit everyone. You'll discover there are many opportunities in everyday life to exercise. You'll find something to motivate you, as it did the ship's crew.

Think of me as your corner-man in the boxing ring – your lifeline – and the ring itself as your new exercise regime. Imagine you are going in the ring for the first time. It's your first bout and I've been training you for months in preparation for this event. We've worked hard to get you disciplined, motivated, focused, *consistent* and confident. I've instilled in you the ability to understand the basics, and to do them well – nothing else. If you can stick to always practising the basics you're on to a winner. If you choose to and are hungry enough to go on and be world champion then good luck to you, but first you have to spend time with me and make sure you soak up all the tips, experience and knowledge I've learnt over the years. Don't run off and find another corner-man if this bout doesn't go how you want it to. Stay committed and slog it out. It will be worth your while. You'll face a few unexpected challenges but as you get a few bouts under your belt it will start to come together. You'll take in what I am passing on to you and you will get a better feel for how it all works *best for you*.

The book is the lifeline you should come back to when the bell rings at the end of each round and you've taken a few knocks. Keep coming back for a break, take on board some good advice, tips and experience, and then get back out in the ring on your own!

All the experience, challenges, high points and low points in your early days will stand you in good stead to move on to other things. It's best to get off to a good start and learn by your experiences, focus on the simple things and do them well. Don't get knocked out in the first round.

A quiet word in your ear...

Before you read on, you need to get your mind set around long-term and consistent exercise no matter what your goals are. That doesn't mean you have to wear lycra and weight-training gloves forever and never dance on tables again. Far from it! Keep an open mind, don't judge yourself and don't stop dancing on tables. If you fail to accept this, I guarantee your success will only be temporary. Don't be demoralised and put off by the thought of a long-term commitment, because if you soak everything up, and do the simple things well, then you'll succeed permanently.

Chapter 1

What is exercise? Why don't you continue to do it?

What does exercise mean to you? What goes through your mind when the word is mentioned? What can it do for you? Why aren't you doing it? If you are doing it occasionally, then why do you keep stopping?

What is exercise?

Everyone's views on exercise are different. They depend on your upbringing, the attitude of the people around you and of course your experiences as a child. You might be lucky enough to be a natural at sport or just have good body co-ordination. It's a genetic lottery. You may not be so lucky. You may feel inferior and have avoided exercise from a young age. Thoughts on what is 'easy' or 'hard' will also differ depending on your experiences, age and ability. But for me exercise is just about getting moving in the most natural and safe way possible, knowing what works for you and making sure you're happy with it. Every professional athlete, serious sportsperson, or average person who enjoys exercising twice a week is doing the same thing. They are getting their whole body moving in the most natural and enjoyable way for them, and they do it *consistently*. If you like to go canoeing, play table tennis, do the gardening, swim, run, lift weights or walk, then that's good enough.

There's a good chance, however, that you haven't got a clue what works for you, and are convinced that there is no form of exercise on this planet that will suit you. But that's probably why you're reading this book. I guarantee that somewhere in here you'll find a form of exercise that's both enjoyable and effective.

Why exercise?

Deep down, most people want to exercise. After all, we know the benefits. Exercise helps strengthen your tendons and ligaments, increases your bone density and improves your heart and lung efficiency. Of course it also helps burn fat, releases natural 'feel-good' chemicals into your body, raises your metabolic rate (which slows as you get older), strengthens your immune system and quite simply makes your body more efficient at living. Who wouldn't want that? Your body is the most complex and amazing thing on this planet. It was built to survive, think, lift and move. Your body needs to exercise. It will last longer, and it will also be kind to you, if you treat it the way it was designed. The best reason to exercise is just to feel good about yourself. We all deserve that.

It may be difficult to contemplate feeling good or enthusiastic about exercise, or even yourself, but that's okay, we're going to change that.

Why don't you exercise?

There are plenty of reasons people don't exercise, and everyone has their own excuses. Everyday life is more sedentary today than it was 20 or 30 years ago, children are less active and there is less physical work required in our normal day. Self-belief is a factor, setting unrealistic goals and hoping for short-term quick fixes will not build your confidence. Deep down you are expecting to fail before you start.

However, the three main reasons people don't exercise are:

Time – life is busy. How can you fit exercise into your life?

You are overwhelmed and just don't know where to start.

You feel uncomfortable and self-conscious when exercising.

Expecting to fail before you start, only thinking about quick fixes, and setting unrealistic goals is an easy way to discourage self-belief.

Once you start, why do you stop?

The most common pattern I see is people throwing themselves into a new fitness and health routine without any realistic thought or long-term planning. New Year's membership of gyms and health clubs has to be the prime example.

Towards the end of each year we are surrounded by the build-up to Christmas, with adverts for presents, meal bookings and special offers to prepare us for the forthcoming onslaught of overindulgence. The fitness campaign goes from infrequent to non-existent around the end of October. By early November dates are being arranged for office parties, family visits, drinks for clients, drinks with customers and mince pies with business associates. We have to write Christmas cards to the whole world, shop in crowded shopping malls, arrange babysitters so we can attend all those parties, and probably meet the bank manager to extend the overdraft. Just when things can't get any worse your neighbours insist you come round for Christmas drinks. You can't refuse – they are your last resort for babysitting. Now, where did I leave my sports kit and trainers?

This may not be an example of everyone's build-up to Christmas, but you can see how the fitness campaign gets lost in the chaos. Without getting involved in an argument about the real meaning of Christmas, it's safe to say that the majority of us lose the plot. But how do you feel after it's all over and you are preparing to get your fitness regime back on track? If you've had an exercise break for a while, January could be a good time to start? The weather will be glorious in the UK in January! Do you feel positive and good about yourself? Probably not...

The trap we often fall into is going from one extreme to the other. If you throw yourself in and get back to exercise three or four times a week after a long break, it will end in tears. If you don't agree, pop into your local gym at 5p.m. on the first Monday in January. It's all doom and gloom – frantic exercisers in new sports kits with the price tags still on. You've just spent the last six weeks partying like Keith Richards of the Rolling Stones, and by the end of January you intend to look like Kate Moss or Brad Pitt. Have a word!

Don't be depressed, slow down to a panic! It's all reversible. Maybe we need to work on some pre-planning, positive thinking and goal-setting.

Hopefully this chapter has made you look at how you think before starting exercise. I'm sure you can relate to at least one of the examples with regards to getting into it all. The reason it's difficult and we keep stopping is because we don't define what we want to achieve. How do you know you've achieved something when you haven't planned what you want in the first place?

Chapter 2

The hardest part is getting changed

Deep down, you already know everything you're going to read in this chapter, but I'm going to lay it all out for you in black and white so it's at the forefront of your mind. Get ready to face some facts.

The basics

If you're still reading, you're probably ready to face some facts:

1. There are no shortcuts, it's got to be a lifelong commitment. Despite what you read and hear, there's no quick-fix, fast-result workout. But you know that anyway, I'm just reminding you.

2. In 25 years' experience as a fitness instructor, I've yet to meet someone who has suddenly started a fitness campaign, gone from no exercise to loads of exercise and kept it up. If you start quickly, you will finish quickly. Fact.

3. Treat exercise like wooing a new love. If you grab hold of them and want to see them four times a week, it will end in tears. See them only now and then, maybe every couple of weeks, and you're probably not really interested. Tease them into your life, welcome them in, have fun when you do, and the chances are it will last. Exercise is the same. You want it to last.

4. Don't worry if you experience some setbacks. You will. Keep your sense of humour, stay frosty, don't take life too seriously and have some faith.

5. It's easy. If you always remember points 1–4 you will succeed.

Throughout the book I will emphasise safe, enjoyable and consistent exercise. These are important points, so just to be clear…

If you want results from exercise it has to be:

- Safe
- Enjoyable
- Consistent

Safe exercise

As far as possible you must be in a risk-free and secure environment. There's always a chance of injuries when exercising, but just use common sense. If you are out running, walking or cycling then be clearly visible to other pedestrians and drivers. If you are in the gym, ensure the equipment is well-maintained and the floor space is clear. Make sure you are dressed in the correct attire for the activity, a decent pair of trainers if you are running, for instance. Chapter 12 deals with before and after exercise and stretching. When you start exercising you will have to suck it and see, and get a feel for it. Begin at a very low intensity and build as the weeks go on. In the early stages try and finish with some energy reserves. Not only will it be safe, it will also build your confidence and enthusiasm as you progress. Don't exercise immediately after a meal; drink water before, during and after exercise. Always listen to the signals from your body.

Enjoyable exercise

Doing exercise that you enjoy most is the key to success. Don't worry what everyone else is doing. If it is an exercise you enjoyed as a kid then you may find it easier than something new and challenging, and therefore it should be safer. If it gets you moving, your body feels warm and your heart rate is up then even better. Get moving in a more dynamic way than usual, and talk and breathe heavily in a sustainable way. This is the equivalent of aerobic (in the presence of oxygen) exercise and is recommended as a good foundation to improve your fitness levels. If you can't think of any exercise you already enjoy, just try a few out. Don't worry about being specific yet – that will come in time – just do something that feels aerobically challenging but still comfortable to you.

Consistent exercise

The *Oxford English Dictionary* describes consistent as 'unchanging' and 'constant'. Don't worry about 'unchanging' – there's a great variety of exercises to keep you interested. Focus on the 'constant' part and you won't go wrong.

But I hate exercise more than anyone in the world!

If you haven't exercised for a while and you're a little out of condition, then it's natural to feel less than excited about exercise. You may have started to think about it in a negative way. You might be reminding yourself of your lack of fitness. The clothes start to get a bit tighter, you are easily out of breath and always lethargic. It's a downward spiral, but a bit like having toothache, you ignore it. Then the ache builds until you are practically screaming at the dental receptionist for an immediate appointment. The dentist pulls your tooth out – pain gone!

It's okay to feel anxious about starting to exercise. Sometimes we just don't want to face up to the fact we're getting older, or that we have let ourselves go and can't do what we did previously. Maybe you finished college a couple of years ago, and are astonished how quickly you've lost your energy and fitness levels. Acceptance is the first step towards changing. Accept that your fitness levels aren't what they once were. Accept that the situation is reversible. Then accept that reversing the situation might take a bit of time. You may be pleasantly surprised, however, to find it's quicker and easier than you think, as well as enjoyable.

Excuses, excuses...

Well, where shall we start? We could talk all day about excuses, and everyone has their own special one. I've heard most of them. The most common one goes something like this:

> 'I've got no time, I'm too unfit, I'm too busy and I'm tired. Anyway, everyone at the gym is really fit, they all know what they are doing and I don't want to look stupid.'

So rather than give you more ideas about excuses, let's change the above excuse into something positive:

You'll start to enjoy exercise so you'll make time for it, therefore you'll get fitter and have more energy. Don't worry about the gym – you can exercise outside. Anyway, you'll be too busy cracking on with your own stuff soon to worry about the fitness freaks. Failing that, I've got plenty of ideas for exercises you can do at home.

'Don't find a fault, find a remedy.'

Henry Ford

How can you afford *not* to exercise? Don't find excuses – you're only cheating yourself. When you get started in the right frame of mind you'll never look back.

It's not what it seems

You've now discovered that you actually don't hate exercise, but are simply hesitant about getting started. Some of you will just dive into the new fitness campaign and crash and burn a few weeks down the line. Some will put it off for as long as possible and then dive in, again and again. It becomes a disaster, similar to someone who tries all different diets, and ends up yo-yo dieting forever.

Your new exercise regime is going to be a slow but sure process. That doesn't mean to say you won't get quick results, but you have to *change your mindset to long term*. If you feel out of condition, you can get positive changes in two weeks if you follow the principles in the book. But we are looking for small, subtle, positive changes that will stay with you, nothing else.

You might think that you have to spend hours in the gym to get your desired results. The thought of it all can just be too overwhelming. But the fact is, *consistency* is far more important than *time spent* exercising. At first, three lots of 10–15 minutes a week spent exercising will be more effective in the long term than two or three weekly one-hour sessions. Try to remember that this is going to last forever. Little and often is good. This way you'll stay enthusiastic and keep your energy up. *Walking away after exercising feeling you could have done more is positive in the early stages.*

Exercise doesn't have to take over your whole life to be effective, but you're going to make slight adjustments to your everyday routine. I see even disciplined exercisers sometimes not get the results they hope for and become very despondent. They might end up stopping altogether or just losing enthusiasm. You just need a tweak here and there to bring in those positive changes. The good news is that you don't have to spend hours and hours in the gym. Just remember *consistency is the key*, then you could get away with a 10-minute workout at home. Deep joy!

Don't be put off by the thought of a long-term approach. Exercise can easily become part of your day and you won't need to stress about it. Before you know it, you'll actually look forward to exercise.

Exercise has to be enjoyable if you want to become disciplined and motivated. Make sure you keep an open mind and be confident that you will soon discover an activity that works for you. You will have to 'woo' it in. It will play hard to get a few times but that's okay, stay frosty and it will soon come running to you.

Personal goals and exercising with your mind

These next chapters will help you plan and think realistically about your goals. Deciding on your aims is personal to you and will be the key to keeping you motivated and helping to feed your self-belief. We will also look at how you think about exercise and get you into a positive mindset to face any new challenges.

Chapter 3

Find a target and don't get distracted

Take a breath and step back

After hard physical exercise at sea as an 18-year-old sailor on a Royal Navy warship, we stopped in Rio. None of the ship's crew had seen a woman for six whole weeks. When that gangway went down, naval discipline was instantly forgotten, local dockyard workers were crushed in the stampede to get to the nearest bar to sample Brazilian beer and practise Portuguese. Like many of the drunken sailors, I fell in love every two seconds, my eyes popped out of my head, I promised marriage and diamond rings, fought, punched and threatened to strangle my shipmates while in hot pursuit, and bought the whole female population of South America expensive cocktails. My brain and sensors had gone into overdrive.

That night we slept either in police cells, in a bin in the dockyard, in a bar or back on the ship alongside the other sailors. Where did it all go horribly wrong?

You can't expect to get everything you want in your life without some prior thinking, planning, groundwork and persistence. If you don't establish what you are aiming for, you won't even realise you have changed your mind!

Don't let your attitude to exercise be like a wet behind the ears sailor going ashore to discover new cultures, bright lights and un-walked paths. Undoubtedly he has bundles of energy, good intentions and enthusiasm, but he also has no firm plan and substance to what he really wants to achieve. If that's the case, your fitness regime will end up like a drunken sailor snoring in a dockyard bin!

Take a breath and step back, think realistically and honestly about what you want in your life. Don't get distracted, overexcited or overwhelmed by other temporary goals that draw you away. Set your goal and focus on it like nothing else matters until you get it.

6Ds – Dave says decide on what you want, delight in every disappointment but don't ever deviate.

Aims and objectives – setting goals

First the bad news. Fitness and health will not come instantly. You can't buy it. It takes time. There are no shortcuts, but there is an easier way.

To be fit and healthy you have to be realistic about what you want to achieve. *No one is physiologically programmed to not benefit from exercise.* Where we go wrong is in setting our goals and fixing the timeframe. You need to sit down and think what you really want, and by when. You could set unrealistic goals, which means you might feel like you've failed. If you're reading this book, you'll probably want to be healthier, burn fat and feel better about yourself. If that's your main goal, make sure you focus on that and don't get distracted. It's okay to be really focused on your goal but it must be in a positive way. It's important not to be motivated by fear of failure, as that could make you anxious and focus in a negative way.

Many of us make exercise more difficult than it actually is, but there is an easier way, *as long as you realise there will be no quick fix, no instant results.* It's a gradual process, something that you have to nurture into your life and your personal circumstances. Don't expect it to fall into your lap without any groundwork. You need to win it over. So take your time, you just need to get a feel for where you're going. It's unfamiliar territory, so follow your instincts and don't take it too seriously. All will come good.

At first you must focus on being *consistent* – any other thoughts are a waste. You know that your fitness and health is reversible. Whatever you do, it has to be *safe, enjoyable* and *consistent.*

Often life's goals are definite and specific, and it's very easy to know when you've achieved them. You might want to learn to ride a bike as a kid, get a degree when you leave school, do an apprenticeship or buy a house. These are all very definite goals, there is no grey area – it is something you want, and you know you can achieve it. These goals might change as you progress, or when you have achieved them you might look for others. Exercise, however, needs a bit more thought and planning. An Olympic athlete like the cyclist Sir Chris Hoy has a definite goal. He knows where he's going, he knows what he wants and he will probably get it. But for the average punter like me and you, defining our goal will take a little more thought.

I've spoken to thousands of people wanting advice on exercise, and when I ask about their goals, most people don't seem to have a definite end result in mind so it often takes a few searching questions. Many will say, 'I want to get rid of this' (the gents generally point to the stomach area, and the ladies point to their hips and thighs). At least, that's the first answer. Then they decide they want to tone up and gain some muscle definition as well. Some people I meet want to run a marathon, walk up Ben Nevis or are hitting 40 and want to feel younger. But I have yet to meet anyone who has instantly come up with a defining target or goal. That's okay – it takes a bit of time and thought, but your goals are for you to decide and they should reflect where you are.

Your own aims and objectives should be SMART!

- Specific. If you want to run the local 5 km fun run then your main focus will eventually have to be running. If you just want to feel better or burn fat then most forms of exercise will get results if you stay consistent.
- Measurable. Can you measure it with a tape measure, training diary, stop-watch, dress size or photograph?
- Achievable. Can you achieve it and enjoy achieving it? Do you really want it and how badly?
- Realistic. Be honest with yourself.
- Time-framed appropriately. Pick a time and date that won't put you under pressure and you will enjoy getting there.

Before you start to exercise, think thoroughly about your goals. Don't worry, nothing will be set in stone and you can change them as you achieve more, but *you* have to decide! Write down your goals on a piece of paper and set them out to last a year. Have a short-, medium- and long-term goal, and an overall goal. Think it through over a couple of days so you can really define what you want. You have to make sure your goals are achievable in the timeframe you have decided. Don't make them so difficult you put yourself under pressure and end up feeling you have failed if you don't meet them. It doesn't have to be anything drastic. 'I want to be more active' is a good enough goal. You are better off setting out something that is easily achievable and building on that, as you'll have a far better chance of consistently achieving your goals. Remember, they will not be set in stone, it will take some time and thought to establish your goals. Don't make the classic mistake of betting your mate £50 you can run a marathon next month as you order your seventh pint of real ale. Your heart has to be in it, you have to do it for *you*, but you must give it some realistic thought. You wouldn't expect an Olympic runner to enter a race and not know where the finish line is! Establish where your finish line will be.

This is a very significant point! Stop and take your time to think. If you don't, it's 'game over, rover'. Don't rush over the gangway without a plan and end up in the dockyard bin!

Overleaf is an example of a client I started working with in March 2004. Sally was in her mid-thirties and had been exercising on an ad hoc basis for a number of years. She was in good health, but had a busy, stressful job that involved a lot of driving around the country.

You could argue some of Sally's goals are a bit vague – 'live a more active and healthy lifestyle' – but they are all measurable and helped get her into the right frame of mind about exercise. There are also some definite goals, i.e. 'Be able to run non-stop for 20 minutes', and can be easily measured. The fact that the goals are broken down and spread out will keep her focused, and also keep up her confidence if she loses a little faith. Each goal is also a little more demanding as it progresses but also achievable. Note there is also no mention of losing weight.

Setting out your goals in this way will be more effective than the £50 bet in the pub, and also better than saying, 'I want to lose this'. As you set out these goals you'll find you make other positive achievements as well – such as losing fat – and these will add to your enthusiasm and self-belief.

It's important to write down your goals and place them in a prominent place – maybe on your fridge, or your diary if you want to be more discreet.

Sally

Sally's overall goals. Start date March 2004

- Live a more active and healthy lifestyle
- Improve general fitness levels
- Improve muscle tone and lose excess body fat
- Make exercise a part of my life

Short-term goals

Start exercising twice a week. Improve heart and lung efficiency and muscular endurance. Be able to run non-stop for 20 minutes by May 2004.

Mid-term goals

Exercise at least three times a week. Improve on fitness levels, to be able to run non-stop for 30 minutes. Eat more healthily and be happier wearing a bikini for holiday in September.

Long-term goals

Exercise four times a week, dropped body-fat percentage to 20 per cent and drop a dress size by March 2005. Exercise is a part of my life.

Read these goals every day, and imagine how good you will feel when you've achieved them.

Be careful of any spoof goals you may have invented. 'I want to run a marathon', 'I'm going to do forward rolls up Mount Snowdon'. You wouldn't believe the promises I hear from some people, when deep down all they want to do is be a bit more healthy and active. There is nothing wrong with aiming to run a marathon, but woo exercise into your life first, *keep it consistent*, and enjoy the fact that each small challenge is part of the journey towards achieving your goal. Then look for other goals and make sure you are hungry to achieve them.

Don't let your head write cheques that your body can't cash! Be honest and realistic with yourself.

Trying to establish your aims and objectives will take a bit of thought. This is where a lot of new exercisers miss out and end up feeling like they may have failed because the plan was not thought through. You have to spend a few quiet moments over a number of days and ask yourself a few questions. Be realistic and honest. Don't be the drunken sailor without any substance or reality in your plan as you run over the gangway! This step is far more important than you may realise. You need to step back and take a breath if you expect to succeed.

Chapter 4

Positive thinking – self-belief

When you've established what you really want from your exercise routine, the next step is to make sure you're thinking about it in a positive way. This chapter will help you to get into a positive frame of mind before you start to exercise. Get that brain and soul to exercise first and your body will join in!

Before I started my course to become a Navy physical trainer I worked in the gym on a shore base and wore the same uniform as the instructors, even though I was not qualified. I was full of myself until an army instructor said I had 'all the gear and no idea'. In my head I went from hero to zero in one second and was instantly having to reassure myself all was good. That was my first lesson in turning a negative thought into a positive thought, and getting the best out of whatever comes your way. It did make me question my ability, but when things got a bit harsh I would work hard to prove him wrong. So I realise he did me a big favour. He didn't know me or my background, and what he said didn't suddenly change who I was, just what I *thought*.

Other people's and your own interpretations are often wrong, so turn their comments *and your own thoughts* into positive thoughts. Get the best out of everything you can.

> 'Thinking is the hardest work there is, which is the probable reason so few engage in it.'
>
> Henry Ford

Hopefully you are reading this book slowly and digesting all these tips to help you succeed. Make sure you gradually lead into these positive thoughts and *consistently* practise them. You have to set out clear aims and objectives for yourself. If there's any doubt, you need to *stop* and *go back* over the last few pages to ensure you are being true to yourself and are clear about what you want.

How can you not benefit from what you are about to achieve? Your goals are attainable and well-planned, and spread out to allow you time to enjoy the new challenge. Your body is designed in such a way that it will benefit from exercise, you are physically capable of doing what you want, it's a win–win situation! You must realise that some days will be tougher than others, you will be pushed to find time and some days miss out on exercise altogether. Don't be too blasé about missing exercise, but don't dwell on it either. Accept it and quickly get back on track.

The next step is just to fill your head with positive thoughts! I recently cycled past the following sign in Bristol:

'*Keep feeding your faith, and your doubts will starve to death.*'

This is how you must think. Everything you ever achieve will start with a thought. Start by being *consistently persistent* about positive thinking and exercise.

It's all about habit and self-discipline. If you have any negative thoughts about exercise then they'll enter your mind naturally and without an invitation. You won't even notice they're there! So you have to really focus and concentrate on thinking positively about exercise and everything else. You have to constantly feed your thoughts of faith, be *persistent* and *consistent*, make it a way of life and stay focused. Watch your mind and thoughts constantly, stay tuned to what is happening in your head and stamp out anything negative. It won't be long before this becomes routine and you'll build your confidence and self-belief. But no one can help – it's down to you and you alone. *You have to help yourself!*

Next time you're carrying out a mundane task, be aware of your thoughts. How much drivel are you churning through over and over again? Start by giving yourself *five minutes a day of total positive exercise thoughts*. You can do it anywhere and at any time, but it has to be a constant five minutes, and it all has to be positive. Do it when you're on the bus, waiting in a queue, washing up, watching the rain, having a shower or doing the ironing. Just find a mundane task and make it worthwhile. When you do it, really imagine yourself being successful at achieving your exercise goal. Just imagine how you'll feel emotionally and physically, and consider all the benefits to you and those around you.

You may find it difficult at first, but persevere with it! Soon it will become easy, and it will affect you and your physical goals in a positive way. Five minutes a day, that's all! As that becomes an easy habit, then start doing it for longer every day. Don't let any negative thoughts enter your head. Stamp them out with totally positive and good emotional thoughts. Then all your mundane tasks become an opportunity for you to mentally prepare yourself for new challenges. You become your own sports psychologist, fitness coach and motivational speaker!

It's important to remember that anything and everything you have achieved has only been done via incremental steps, whether it's riding a bike, learning a new language or getting a new job. The things you really want always take a bit of work and patience. Often the waiting to get started is the most difficult part. You have to take little steps each day. As soon as you wake focus on what you are going to achieve.

Free beer and chocolate ice cream forever!

Okay, I'm telling a lie, but I needed to get your attention somehow. If I'd written 'visualisation' then the majority of you would have skipped the whole paragraph! Now as far as I'm concerned you're doing this 'visualisation' thing already, but not necessarily in an effective way. What's going through your mind when you think about exercise? You could be visualising something negative that will make you even more anxious. Maybe it gives you a positive and exciting feeling.

When you are planning a holiday, buying a new car, going to university or a job interview, getting married, getting divorced or having a baby, you are visualising the event. It's in our nature to imagine future events, regardless of whether we perceive them to be good or bad. If you're saving up for a new sports car, you can see yourself in it, smell the leather seats and hear the engine. Think back to the times you have had similar thoughts.

Now, consider how your thought processes and feelings have been leading up to exercise. Even if you've always done exercise, consider how you feel about it after a break or illness. If your thoughts are totally positive, great, you're on your way. But if you consider past failings in a negative way, how is it going to feel after a long layoff? You need to have a word and change your thoughts.

Regardless of where you are on your fitness campaign you need to start thinking, dreaming and imagining in a positive way.

> 'Champions aren't made in gyms. Champions are made from something they have deep inside them. A desire, a dream, a vision.'
>
> Muhammad Ali

If it's good enough for an Olympic athlete or professional sportsperson then it's good enough for you. The difference is that athletes have probably been doing what they do since they were very young. Their talent was spotted at an early age and their coaches, friends and family have encouraged them and told them they are the best. Why not? They probably are a bit special, and this positive environment has encouraged their self-belief. Still, to get that extra edge over their opponents they'll have a sports psychologist to enhance their confidence and help them keep a strong mind.

Not everyone has the time and money to employ an expert just to tell them they're great. Don't worry, you don't need to, you can do it yourself. As you regularly practise your five minutes a day of positive thoughts, and go about your everyday life you're also going to visualise. It's up to you what you visualise, but I recommend you relate it to the aims and objectives you have just established. For instance, if your goal is to run the local 10 km road race then visualise that. I don't just mean imagine running around the block. Go through all of it in your head: the journey there, the smells, the physical challenge, the sounds, the atmosphere and the feeling of success on completion. Imagine your work colleagues, family and friends congratulating you. Go through the whole process in your mind. The more you practise the easier it gets, and it will have an encouraging effect on your physical goals. Again, if anything negative starts to creep in, stamp it out and quickly change it to a good thought.

Visualise your success – seeing is believing.

'Failing to prepare, means you are preparing to fail.'

Abraham Lincoln

You have to prepare yourself in your mind if you really want to make those changes. Miss this bit out, and there's a very good chance you'll stop for so long you'll have to go through the process again – and again. *Get into it now! Don't dismiss the value of visualisation!*

Change how you think, feel and see exercise. Visualise in only a positive way. It takes time and practice, but it works wonders. Imagine your success. If you stick at it you'll eventually shift your mind until your thoughts become a reality. *Be persistently consistent, and consistently persistent* – and you will succeed.

You can apply the visualisation process to any of your goals. You could imagine wearing a size 10 dress rather than a 14, or imagine fitting into your old favourite suit and how good that would make you feel. One of my clients completed the *Marathon des Sables* in the Sahara Desert in March 2008. For training, every Friday for two years we ran for an hour at 6 a.m. As we approached the end he would go quiet and imagine he was running in the desert towards the finish line after 200 km over seven days in temperatures of 100 degrees. Now, try and do that in Bristol in December! It takes some imagination, concentration and being *persistently consistent*. It worked for my client. As the weeks went on he found it easier to focus his mind, and when it got emotional in the desert he just cracked on. He did the race in his head first, and his body joined in.

'The ancestor of every action is a thought.'

Ralph Waldo Emerson

Be focused – all the time

Imagine it. Feel it. But only in a totally positive way! It can be challenging to think positive if you don't feel positive, but it will become easier the more you do it. There is no other way. Any other thoughts are pointless. There is absolutely *no room whatsoever for negative thoughts*. You'll never achieve anything if you don't either believe you can do it, or trick yourself into believing you can. Don't even think about starting to exercise until your mind is doing it first.

Get your mind to start exercising, and your body will join in

It will all come good, and you'll trick the negative part of your imagination. Be more positive than you have ever been in your life. Be focused, concentrate and have some faith in yourself.

I've met plenty of good sportspeople who don't bother with any visualisation. They are quite happy to chuck themselves around the gym or run for an hour most evenings after work without even thinking about it. It's ingrained into them, it's all they know and they are happy to do that. I've also seen them when they're forced to stop. Even if it's only for a week or two – because of an injury, for example – they become anxious that they'll lose their fitness gains. This is a good example of negative visualisation. This doesn't happen to everyone, but some people get irritable or moody, mentally tired or stressed if they miss their exercise fix. I know people who've become depressed because they have to stop their regular exercise.

Everyone can benefit from a little positive visualisation.

Motivation

Dictionary definitions of 'motivate' and 'motivated' include the phrases 'incentive to', 'stimulate the interest of, inspire' and 'having a definite and positive desire to do things'. You may not associate words 'stimulate', 'interest', 'definite', 'positive' and 'desire' with exercise. However, having got this far, you should be confident that you can stimulate your own desires and achieve your definite goals.

It's natural at first to be cynical about your ability to achieve your goals, but you're going to have to be *persistently consistent* when it comes to keeping your faith. Motivation is something that only you have control of, only you can control your mind and your thoughts. You may have some expert advice around you – a personal trainer or a training buddy – and that's good. But the buck stops with you. *You are responsible* for your own motivation. Instead of a New Year's resolution that may fade in February, have a New Day resolution, just a simple one that lasts 365 days! Say it and do it every morning.

Saying something out loud will make you focus. I'm not advising you to shout your goal for the day at the top of your voice on the train, but saying something will make you forget any other thoughts. It only takes a few seconds.

I see some of my clients for one hour a week. There are 168 hours in a week, so what will you do for the other 167 hours?

There are plenty of motivational tricks in the following chapters. Some will jump out and help you along the way, but you have to get a good base from which to work. It all comes down to planning your goals, giving yourself the time you need and staying focused. I have had experience working with Olympic athletes, professional and semi-professional sportspeople, hardened and highly motivated servicemen

Micky

Micky was in his mid-forties, in reasonable shape and in good health. He had a busy management job that involved long hours and travelling around the south-west of England. He enjoyed exercise but complained he wasn't seeing any improvements in his fitness levels. Micky enjoyed going to the gym once a week, and would spend over an hour exercising, usually a bit of running, cycling and some free weights. He complained that he could only run for about 1 km before he had to walk, but his goal was to run 6 km without stopping.

There was a simple remedy to Micky's training programme. At the start, his routine was a bit haphazard and he was trying to cram everything into one session a week. However, the good point was that he was *consistent* and enjoyed what he was doing. As his main goal was to run 6 km without stopping we focused on his running for six weeks. We shortened his gym time from about 70 minutes to 30 minutes, but got him to exercise three times a week. This obviously took a little more commitment and planning, but the idea was to make the sessions shorter, more focused, more enjoyable and a lot more effective. All we did was to get Micky to do 'Dave's 'Simple but Special' (see page 99). This consisted of one minute walking and one minute running for 20 minutes, building on the length of running time per session.

Within two weeks he was astounded at how far and for how long he could run. He quickly got to grips with his pace judgement, his confidence and enthusiasm soared as he could see improvements. The sessions became a lot more effective, so he felt more energised and motivated. Before long Micky's stamina and distance improved, and he could soon comfortably run 6 km.

in the Special Forces, gym junkies, not-so gym junkies and exercise avoiders! I promise you that everyone from Olympic athletes down has bad days, days when it's all going wrong, you feel cranky, heavy and your body just doesn't want to join in. These days often arrive when there's free beer and chips at your local pub to test your motivation!

Bad days

Once you get it into your head that bad days are normal, it will be a bit easier. You'll be able to deal with them better. *Bad days are good* – they make you appreciate the good days even more!

There are plenty of reasons for a bad day. You might be genuinely tired, ill, overtraining or just bored. The important thing is to recognise when you are stuck and figure out why you feel unmotivated. I'd go so far as to say that the sooner you have a bad day the better! The sooner it comes along, the sooner you'll learn to recognise it, deal with it and turn it into an opportunity. As you exercise more, your bad days will be become less frequent and good days will become the norm.

> 'Self belief is required to become a champion. To achieve this you must become a champion of self belief.'

> Anonymous

Don't let anyone change your mind

During my resettlement time leaving the Royal Navy I took a flight to Cape Town for a bit of a break. I only had a few weeks until I would be a fully fledged ex-matelot and full-time civvy! I was a bit anxious going from a secure job for 22 years to working for myself – back to wearing shorts and hoovering treadmills at 40 years of age! I ended up chatting to an ex-soldier on the flight and was keen to pick his brains about making the transition to civvy street. He was an ex-military policeman with about 30 years' service and now exported fish from Norway to South Africa, and South African wine back to Europe. What a lifestyle change! He only said a few words. 'Mate, take your time to decide what you want to do. Once you've done that don't let anyone change your mind.'

Be honest with yourself about what you want to achieve, make sure it's attainable and give yourself some time. Be patient when working out your goals. They should affect you and those around you in a constructive way. When you've decided, sit on that thought for a few days and build up your self-belief with plenty of positive thinking. Visualise so much you start to get on your own nerves! Then do it some more. Be persistent and laugh at the setbacks when they come (because they will), and if you stay persistent, when you least expect it, it will fall into your lap.

Chapter 5

Keep the target in your sights consistently and persistently

Now that you've established your goals and have confidence that you can achieve them, you need to keep feeding your faith and stay positive. This chapter will help to keep you motivated, but it will also give you a heads-up about the challenges that can nudge you off track. I'm going to talk about habit-forming and the importance of being patient as you move forward, keep improving and become more aware and self-reliant about exercise.

Habit-forming

Consistency is the key to everything in life. It doesn't matter if you've discovered the perfect training routine, if you're not *consistent* it won't work. There's absolutely no point in wasting energy training hard, but not *consistently*. You're better off exercising more frequently at a lower intensity. You might find the results come more slowly, but they'll stay with you. Those small, subtle changes will gather momentum. As you continue to get better at visualising you'll naturally become more focused and positive.

Slow but sure – haste makes waste

Once you've accepted that you can exercise forever, you'll need to keep everything simple and be patient! You're going to find the exercise that you most enjoy. At first, don't worry about the effectiveness of what you are going to do. If your body is out of condition, or you've not taken part in exercise on a regular basis for a while, then two sessions of 20 minutes this week is more than you did last week. It's a step in the right direction.

In the world today we can get most things instantly – food, money, clothes, a new car, a house. It can be easy for some and not others. But your health and fitness? There are no shortcuts for anyone. Be patient, enjoy what you do and you'll be pleasantly surprised at the results you can achieve

Commitment

This is obviously very important if you want to achieve anything, but you won't stay committed if you haven't really established what it is you're trying to commit to! The previous chapters are very important, and if you haven't grasped the importance of the main points so far then there's no point reading any further. You are now committing yourself to consistently exercising for the rest of your life. There is simply no other way, and no point. Now before you launch this book out of the window, you have to believe me – it's not as bad as it sounds as long as you plan properly, woo exercise in and stay consistent.

I read an article about England rugby player Jonny Wilkinson, in which he talked about commitment and motivation. His strength and conditioning coach Steve Black had plenty of good ideas about commitment. He would get Wilkinson to imagine someone had been videoing him all day and then go through his day in his head at night. This gave him the opportunity to ask himself if he was happy with his day and if he was doing himself and his team members justice. Wilkinson is undoubtedly a highly motivated and committed athlete who will always look to get the best results, and we can learn from his methods. If you're going to commit yourself to exercising from now on, how will you feel as you watch over the day's events before you go to bed? You may do this already without even realising it. If you're going to think about how your day has gone or how tomorrow will be, make sure it is as positive as can be. This is not a chance to beat yourself up, but a few minutes at the end of the day to ask if you've done the best for yourself. It's a very good way of getting focused and committed. It will get easier the more you do it and can produce very good results.

Genuine challenges to be aware of and prepared for

Even though you've established your aims and objectives, and are persistently thinking positive, unexpected challenges will present themselves. This chapter will help you to expect the unexpected, keep your goals in mind and stay focused. Very often in life things that we expect to be difficult turn out to be easier than we thought. The opposite can sometimes be the case: a challenge that we think is insignificant can turn out to be tougher than we imagined.

There are many situations that prevent us integrating exercise into our daily routine and many simple ways to get around them. *Which one of these excuses is yours?*

Time

Time is always the biggest excuse. For this reason it's important to start off with short and easy-to-arrange bouts of exercise. A 30-minute workout could end up taking two hours from your day if you have to travel to and from the gym and find a parking space. Plan your exercise around your day. Other things will crop up to give you lots of excuses not to exercise, which is why I'm a big fan of exercising before your normal day starts. Then it's done, over. It should be comforting to know that there are simple ways to nurture your exercise routine into your everyday life. Just don't get overwhelmed by the thought of it all. Stay focused, be positive, you'll eventually find time because you want to do it.

Logistics

Planning your exercise will help you find time. I bet before you have a big night out with your mates you'll plan it as well as any military commander about to go to war! So do the same when you think about the next day's bout of exercise. Just a couple of minutes' thought and preparation will save time and ensure it happens, and will also mentally prepare you for it! Simple things like just getting your sports kit out and putting it in a prominent place will work. 'I can't find my kit' is an unworthy excuse as you rush out to work with toast crumbs all over your chin. It's very common for people to struggle in the early stages when trying to find a routine. *This is a bigger hurdle than you realise.* Doing the exercise is the fun, easy and enjoyable bit!

I spent six months training to be a Royal Navy physical training instructor. The course was arduous, long, very physical and it just took over your life. We would be up at 5 a.m. and work on average until midnight. Our instructor, a Royal Marine sergeant had a favourite saying: 6 Ps. 'Prior preparation prevents piss-poor performance'. He was spot on. When we didn't plan our work it all went wrong. It stuck out if we weren't focused, thinking and planning what we were supposed to be doing, and we knew it. So get into that habit, plan ahead, make it happen.

Family

Starting an exercise programme will eat into your already busy life and may affect your relationship with your parents, partner or children. Everyone wants a piece of you, so discuss your plans with those close to you before you start. They need to realise how important it is to you to succeed, and you'll need each other's support and patience. But whatever you do don't feel guilty. We are all entitled to time to ourselves, and if approached properly this could benefit all parties.

Work

If you spend 40 hours a week at work it's going to have an effect on your exercise regime. You'll need to put even more thought into the planning stages. Exercise will help you de-stress and relax, but it will need to be well balanced with your working week. Start with short, easy sessions that won't tire you out and build on that.

Cost

Be wary of joining a gym and signing up for a yearly membership thinking the expense will make you go. This is rarely the case. Start somewhere you can pay as you go. Positive thinking, visualisation and exercising in your head will cost nothing, and if you practise that thoroughly it will save you time, cost and effort in the long run. Or just buy some decent trainers and get out in the fresh air. It's free!

Exercise – is it constructive or destructive?

Initially, it will take some time to nurture your new routine into your life. It might seem a bit destructive, especially when you find it difficult to get motivated, and normal life just gets in the way. Don't worry, any new challenge is the same. Exercise may make you feel tired to begin with but that will pass and you'll soon have more energy after exercising. If you've taken on board all the information from the previous chapters you should by now be in a positive frame of mind and well prepared to succeed at this challenge. Take your time, be realistic and recognise it will take some persistence to get used to your new ways. Go back to the beginning of the book again, and read the first five points on exercise. Welcome it into your life, and it will soon be constructive for you and those around you.

The Rock

I have a friend who I served with in the Navy – we were on physical training instructors aptitude where he took me under his wing. His nickname in the Navy was 'The Rock'. That's what he was: hard as granite and the most reliable mate ever. At the start of his career he was repeatedly told that he would never be a PTI and was told to go back to his ship and not darken the doors of the Navy PT school ever again. But nothing could stop The Rock. I have never met anyone so determined – he kept going back for more and more. He never moaned or disputed anyone's decision, he just dug deeper and deeper and tried even harder. He was a fabulous PT instructor and is now a fireman. He might not have had the sporting ability of others, but he made up for it with sheer commitment, hard work and determination. We all have a bit of that to call on somewhere.

You should be more aware now that exercising is only a small part of a bigger plan. To maintain your regime you'll sometimes feel like you're spinning plates on sticks. Each plate is a representation of all the other responsibilities in your life – family, work, social life, education, partners and of course rest and relaxation. You could make the classic schoolboy error of just spinning one or two plates, but then it's only a matter of time before the rest come smashing to the ground. Give equal attention to all the plates and keep them spinning all the time.

What's the point reading this book and not carrying out any action now? Why start tomorrow, next week or next year? The fact you are reading this book proves that you want to make some changes and already are doing something about it! Be pleased with yourself and make the next move. Now is as good a day to start as any. The easiest option is often the wrong option.

The sooner you start, the sooner you finish.

> 'Exercise in the morning before your day starts. It's like being 1 – 0 up at half time.'
>
> Mike Daly, personal trainer

Chapter 6

Exercise – it's all about you

Your goals have now been set out, and you know they're going to fit your lifestyle. It's okay to listen to what other exercisers are doing, but what works for them will not necessarily work for you. Be confident that in the next chapter you can establish the best way to come out of the starting blocks, start slowly and build on your routine and fitness gains.

What's best for me?
By now you will have established clearer goals, and know when and how you're going to achieve them. What's best for you is specific to your own personal objective. It's very difficult to achieve anything if you don't enjoy what you do, so what's best for you is something that is both enjoyable and safe. You don't need to understand and know everything about exercise, all the ins and outs. Work to discover what will be easy for you and fit into your life. You will still have to organise and plan, but just do the basics well and often. If the exercise you plan to do is *safe* and *enjoyable* then the next stage is to ensure you are *consistent*.

'It's their Olympic Games, their World Cup Final!'
This was a favourite saying of a senior instructor I once worked for. He had coached at national and Olympic level and was a very hard but fair taskmaster. He believed in treating all exercisers and sportsmen/women the same. They are all out there having a go, giving it their best shot every time and that's all that matters. Make it your own Olympic Games.

If you haven't exercised for a while then you definitely don't need to be too regimented in the exercise programme you follow. The more functional the better. Exercises such as walking, running and using your own bodyweight as resistance works. Exercises such as squats, planks, hip raises and press-ups (see the Six for Life exercises on page 78) are both challenging and good for all-round conditioning, but doing what you enjoy is more important for now. Anything that gets you moving and increases your heart rate will be beneficial, and will also give you a good foundation for moving on to more challenging and focused work.

It's important to remember that *consistency* should come before specificity. So try and find the easiest and most practical form of exercise and fit it into your normal routine, ensuring it causes minimum stress. There is no rush, be patient. You might be chomping at the bit to get started, but try a few different forms of exercise that appeal to you. Don't run if you don't like running. Forget what everyone else is doing – the early stage is a fun and exciting place to be, so just enjoy the freedom of doing exercise that feels natural.

How long should I exercise for?
Anywhere between 10 and 40 minutes when you first start will be okay depending on how long you've been away from exercise. It doesn't matter in the first few weeks, *consistency* overrides everything else. If the first week consists of three bouts of exercise lasting 10 minutes, 30 minutes and 15 minutes, that's great. You've achieved three sessions in a week – which is consistent and achievable. As you continue you'll get a feel for how long you can exercise for. At first you may get tired, but your stamina will improve and you'll recover quicker. If you're sticking with *safe*, *enjoyable* and *consistent* exercise then after a few weeks you'll maintain a higher level of intensity, so working for 20–30 minutes will get results.

How often should I exercise?
How often can you exercise in a week and keep it up forever? That may sound daunting, but it can be easily achieved as long as you woo in your new exercise regime. It's far better to exercise once a week and maintain that for a while before moving up to twice a week, than to promise yourself you'll exercise four times a week and only do it twice. If you aim to exercise twice a week and end up training three times, then even better!

Be careful not to set your sights too high. Make your goals achievable and build on that. In a perfect world you would be exercising three or four times a week, but we don't live in a perfect world, and there's no one size fits all answer. *Consistency* is the key. It has to be a gradual process. I've yet to meet someone who has suddenly started exercising four times a week and kept it up. Enthusiasm is all well and good, but *keep it in a jar, unscrew the cap and use up a little at a time*. If you let it all out at once it will disappear and you can't borrow anyone else's.

If you think along these lines and stay consistent with your weekly goals it will be easier to keep exercising. Most people have busy lives, so organisation and realistic weekly exercise plans are a deciding factor in the end result.

By now any negative thoughts about spending hours in the gym should have disappeared. You might be a bit cynical about the benefits of a 10-minute workout, but I'm speaking from experience. Those short workouts are the key to keeping you consistent and achieving your goals. You don't bury an acorn in your back garden and expect a monstrous oak to appear the next day!

Challenges, mistakes and making exercise easy

The next section will help highlight a few common mistakes when it comes to exercising and also how to face challenges that may crop up. You may be able to relate to a few of the examples. After these chapters you will be able to 'step back' and ensure your fitness campaign is on track.

Chapter 7

Tricks of the trade

This chapter highlights a few little tricks and practical ways of maintaining your fitness regime. I picked these up just by watching other exercisers and experimenting myself. Although there are no shortcuts, the routines in this section will keep you on a more direct path to your goals. One thing, though – don't suddenly try all the tips and routines; soak them up and keep them in mind as you progress. Keep coming back to this chapter when you feel the need, or when you want to reassess your routine.

Ten top tips

1. Don't get sucked into the belief that you have to workout for 40 minutes or more every time you exercise. If you're pushed for time and only have a free 10 minutes, just exercise for 10 minutes. But raise the tempo, work a lot harder than you would for 30 or 40 minutes. It's definitely worth it. Say you miss 20 workouts a year because of time, perhaps five of those are genuine, but the other 15 are just excuses. Swap those 15 weak excuses for 15 10-minute workouts. They'll keep you consistent and your body will start to expect it and adapt to it in a positive way.

2. Gear before beer. Plan the next day before you wind down. If you're exercising in the morning then leave your workout kit next to your bed and put it on as soon as you wake. Decision made. That means before you sleep you are mentally preparing to work out tomorrow. If you know you'll hear the alarm in the morning and hit the snooze button, sleep in your sports kit!

3. Food. It's also important to plan what you are going to eat the following day. Remember – exercise is the easy part, it's all the other logistics that stop you exercising. Get into a routine of planning your fuel for the next day. If you're going to exercise before work, make sure you have some food ready to eat after you've worked out, before you go into that early board meeting. The same applies if you are exercising at lunchtime. You won't have time to queue in the canteen or the local sandwich shop if you've been for a long walk. If you're exercising after work, make sure your energy levels are kept up with plenty of water and an afternoon snack. It might be a pain to think, plan and prepare for the next day in this way, but if you neglect this part of your exercise routine it will grind to a halt. Remember the '6 Ps'. You don't have to spend hours preparing, just a quick 10 minutes, and make sure you take it into account when you go food shopping. It'll soon become as much a part of your routine as the exercise itself!

4. If you exercise three or four days a week every evening after work and want to switch to exercising in the morning, do it gradually so your body clock has time to adjust. Just work out in the morning once a week, and train at the normal time for the rest of the week. Over a period of a few weeks, start training in the morning twice a week and increase the frequency until morning exercise becomes normal.

5. Listen to your body. When you're feeling tired, ease off or rest – your body tells you everything you need to know. Injuries, tiredness and illness are normally your body's way of telling you to take it easy, that it needs to recuperate – so don't fight it. It's important to be honest, though, and don't confuse lethargy, laziness or lack of discipline with a genuine need to take a break.

6. Don't beat yourself up if you miss a session or go away on holiday. And don't try to make up the time by cramming in more sessions in a week than you're used to. Make sure the first couple of sessions back are light and less intensive than before your break. You might feel a bit lethargic after your time away, but your body hasn't forgotten how to exercise. Just stay focused

and remember that to achieve long-term, consistent results it's best to be patient. However, a good way to avoid this stress is to…

7. … Exercise on holiday. This might sound extreme or obsessive, but it doesn't need to be. Let's face it – the biggest excuse for not exercising is time. You have plenty of free time on holiday, and therefore no excuses! This doesn't mean you have to join the local gym and spend hours exercising. You only need to do 10 minutes a day. Even if that's a significant drop from your normal routine it will still be worthwhile. It doesn't have to be a structured or regimented programme, just something to get you moving. A walk or a jog is perfect; a challenging swim in the hotel pool or basic bodyweight exercises such as planks, press-ups and squats will be enough. The most important thing is that you do *something*. I guarantee it will be so much easier when you return to real life. Having decided to exercise on holiday, make sure you do something within the first 24 hours of arriving – otherwise it won't happen. It's crucial to get into that routine straight away. If you are lucky enough to be taking a break for two or three weeks, it's no good deciding to exercise towards the end of your holiday. This may not seem practical if you're on a coach tour, a cruise or safari, but there's always 10 minutes in the day to make time for yourself. Trust me, if you've done a bit of exercise, your cold beer or ice cream will taste even better!

8. If there's an exercise that you find really challenging and want to improve, then do it every day for 10–14 days. An exercise that just requires your own body weight – such as squats or press-ups – is perfect. Find a point that you walk past frequently every day and do your challenging exercise every time you pass that point. For instance, every time you walk through your kitchen door, do 6–12 press-ups. You'll be astounded at how much you improve over the 10 days.

9. No matter how much you enjoy exercise, there will always be days when you feel lethargic and don't want to do it. Before forcing yourself, make sure you're not ill, overdoing it or your body is telling you to rest for a genuine reason. If you're used to

exercising for an hour but just can't face it, then knock 75 per cent off the time of your workout. That leaves you 15 minutes to exercise, so give yourself five minutes to warm up and prepare properly. Once the warm-up is complete, then just go crazy and see how much you can achieve in 15 minutes. Increase the intensity and work rate, but make sure you stop and cool down after 15 minutes. Don't do this all the time – it's not an excuse – but sometimes you can get away with it. You'll feel good afterwards, and you'll still have 45 minutes spare. Just be aware the first time this happens that it's important to listen to your body and tune in to its responses!

10. Unless you are ill, injured or genuinely tired you will never regret *doing* some form of exercise, but you will probably regret *not* doing it. *Think how you will feel after and not before.*

The easiest part of an exercise regime is the exercise itself. It's all the other things going on in your life that make it seem impractical. The 'tricks of the trade' are mostly common sense, and after a bit of experience you'll conjure up your own ways of working towards your goal, and then you will find it fits easily into your life and routine.

> 'No matter what amount of work you have, you should always find time for exercise, just as you do for your meals. It is my humble opinion that, far from taking away from one's capacity for work, it adds to it.'
>
> M. K. Gandhi

Chapter 8

Unfamiliar and unexpected challenges

'Round again coxswain'

Steering a small inflatable boat alongside a warship can be daunting at times, especially in a rough sea with a few shipmates leaning over the guardrails hoping for some entertainment at your less-than-efficient driving skills! Well, everyone on board is rooting for you when you're on your way back from the supply ship with the mail. As you line up your approach, and the waves are smashing you against the ship's side, you sense that the fighting efficiency of the crew rests with you and not the commanding officer. Having to face a tattooed chief stoker after dumping his Valentine cards at the bottom of the North Sea is not a way of making life at sea pleasant. Get it wrong, and the shout from the chief bosun's mate 'Round again coxswain!' won't build your street credibility with the eyes watching you either. So don't be a 'round again coxswain' on your fitness campaign. You'll get nudged against the ship's side a few times, and probably dump the chief stoker's love letters, but don't jump overboard just yet. It's only a matter of time until you're taking the lads ashore for a barbecue in the Seychelles!

The following questions have been compiled from the last 25 years of working in an exercise environment. They are common questions asked by people about to embark on an exercise programme. Which ones apply to you?

I'm desperate to change my body shape. I'm going to join the gym, but I know I won't like it.

Change your thinking. You are focusing on the negative. You expect to feel intimidated by the people and the equipment, and are worried that everyone is looking at you. Go back to the chapter on positive thinking and reinforce it as many times as you need to. There are alternatives to exercising at the gym – outside or in your home – but we can talk about that later. At this stage, positive thinking is more important than anything, and where you exercise is less important than how you *feel* about exercise.

You talk about self-motivation. I've not done any exercise for 10 years! How can I get motivated?

How can you afford not to? Your body has been designed to think, walk, lift, jump and run. If you don't start now, nothing will change. Your body has been used to not exercising, so now let it get used to exercise. Go back to the start of the book. Tell yourself you can do it. Believe you can.

But I'm always tired! I've got no time!

You're probably not tired, just lethargic. Once you start you won't regret it. You'll quickly get more comfortable with your work rate and pace judgement as you 'feel' your way in. Then you'll see how much energy you really have, how your sleep improves, how you can concentrate more, how your self-esteem and confidence grow. Swap that for feeling tired.

I hate exercise, I always have, it's pointless!

Okay, don't exercise then. Go back and sit on the couch, turn on the TV, open a big bag of crisps and a can of beer. Then tell me how you feel! It's never too late, but the later you start, the harder it will be to get into condition. The longer you leave it, the more your body will get used to doing nothing. It will be inefficient at living. Grab the chance to add a few years to your life. When you exercise, things around you will start to change. You'll feel better inside and out, sleep better, be more confident, think more efficiently, eat better, laugh more and generally be a lot happier. Start now!

Everyone will laugh at me!

Everyone will be too busy getting on with their own stuff to worry about you so forget it. No one else is in a position to comment on what you are doing, so just get amongst it!

I feel rubbish!

It's all in your mind. The sooner you start exercising today, the sooner you finish. When you come home, just go out and walk in the fresh air for 20 minutes. Once your exercise is done, maybe eat some healthy food and drink lots of water. Sit down and relax, give yourself a bit of time out, tell yourself you feel good.

There's no way I can go to the gym after work. No time.

Okay, fair enough. Just figure out when will be the *least* difficult time to go. Start by getting up 10 minutes earlier, and do some light exercise in the morning – just a 10-minute walk around the block. You have to start somewhere, and I'm afraid you have to be patient. You *can* do it, but you have to be positive, and you have to want it. Don't let little obstacles sap your energy and put you off.

I still feel fat!

'I've been exercising for three weeks now. It's great. I have loads of energy, I'm sleeping better and I feel really good about myself. But when I look in the mirror, nothing's changed. The scales are the same and I still feel fat!'

Slow down to a panic. It's very, very early. Look at all the positives you've just mentioned. Think about how it's making you feel, the satisfaction and buzz after exercise. Focus on that feeling for now. Let your body adapt slowly. Things are happening that you can't see. Can you exercise for longer now than you could two weeks ago? Of course you can. Your heart is getting stronger, your lung capacity is improving, your tendons and ligaments are stronger. Your body is becoming more efficient at living. Go with it. As for the scales. Throw them away. Give them to someone you don't like. Sell them on eBay. Your body is more likely to be increasing in muscle tone due to the increase in exercise, so your metabolic rate has increased and your body is more effective at burning fat. The scales are not telling the whole truth. Go by how you feel and how your clothes fit. Have some faith!

I've been exercising for three months. I love it, but I'm stuck in a rut. I had loads of positive changes at first and now nothing.

Don't worry – that's normal. Your body has become tolerant to exercise, and adaptations will get a little more challenging. This is a crucial time, and the point at which you can get frustrated. Watch for the signs. Are you less enthusiastic about exercise, or do you go straight home from work rather than to the gym? If the answer is 'yes', don't worry; there may be many reasons for this. It's difficult when the speed of results slows down. You need to reassess your goals and get some new ideas. There are plenty of simple tricks to get you revitalised, but you need to do them now. Recognise where you are and take some advice. Just a small change will work.

My exercise programme is going well, but every so often I have a rubbish session, and just can't do it.

That's okay. It's good to have a session like that sometimes – then you appreciate the good ones! Maybe you've been doing too much, no doubt there are other things going on in your life. Don't stress, your body will look after you, just listen to it and accept the fact you might be tired. You haven't failed. Tiredness is only temporary, so rest if you have to.

I want to get fit, so I'm going to run a half marathon, or maybe start playing football or squash.

That's cool, not a problem, but slow down. Do some form of steady state – aerobic (i.e. being able to talk in-between breaths) general fitness before taking part in a contact team sport, or something as dynamic as squash. Lots of twisting, lunging and jumping might be a bit much if you're out of condition. Get fit to play sport rather than play sport to get fit. The same applies to entering something like a half marathon – lots of enthusiasm in the early stages, but sometimes it can be too much. Once the event is over it's easy to slip back to where you were before, and difficult to get started again. Consistency is the key.

I don't know what to do!

'My mate says try this programme, do this training. Mr Celebrity swears by his new exercise regime; Miss Celebrity says "do this", "eat this", "do these exercises". I don't know what to do!'

Who cares what everyone else is doing? It doesn't matter. Ask yourself, 'Can I do it for life?' Will it be easy to maintain forever, just with a few small adjustments as you get a bit older? Are the principles simple and will they be easy to keep as part of your life? *Your life*! It's all about you. Forget everyone else, stick to the simple principles and it will work. We all know the answers, we just need reminding. You *can* exercise consistently, vary what you do, lay off the fats, eat a balanced and colourful diet. It's do-able.

The previous points seem to be common with many people I've worked with and easy to spot if you just take a step back and evaluate where you are. Another challenge may not be obvious and can sometimes catch many exercisers out regardless of experience…

The plateau

The plateau is something all exercisers should be aware of. You may not experience it in the early stages of your exercise programme, but it will definitely sneak up on you at some point. It quietly follows you around for days and you don't even notice it's there. It watches you, your habits and routine. It waits until you are tired, vulnerable and your defences are weak. Then – bang! It's game over. So, keep a lookout, concentrate on how you are feeling and do the simple things well. Soon it'll go and find someone else to bother.

The plateau stage can be physical as well as mental. As you start an exercise routine your body will find it challenging but will quickly adapt. Depending on your physical make-up, health and age, your rate of improvement will vary. Seasoned athletes take a scientific approach to their schedule, sports scientists and conditioners plan a programme to last four years with the intention of the athlete reaching their peak at the Olympic Games, for instance. These experts prepare for their athletes' bodies to plateau, and ensure they have enough time to rest, recover and move on. Each sportsperson is different, but most undertake some sort of 'active recovery' week when their body needs a rest. They won't sit around drinking beer and eating pies for a week, but they will ease off the intensity, stay active, eat healthily and make a few subtle changes for a short time.

Take a similar action with your own routine. If you like to stick to the same routine at the same time and it works for you, then have a week of change every 6–8 weeks. If you're happy just cracking on with no specific routine then that's okay too, as long as it's working for you. Whatever sort of exerciser you are, you will hit a plateau. It's not a major concern, it's just your body warning you that you need to rest or vary what you're doing.

You'll start to feel good as soon as you maintain and enjoy exercise. In the early stages the improvements come quickly – you can see and feel the changes within a few weeks. If your family, friends or work colleagues notice and compliment you, your enthusiasm and determination will grow. The encouragement will keep you enthused and you may work harder to achieve more changes. Your body will respond by becoming more tolerant to exercise – and that's when you start to plateau. Compared to the initial changes to your muscle tone and body shape, it will feel difficult to achieve more. Your enthusiasm may dip; it becomes too tempting just to press the snooze button on the alarm, to accidentally forget to pack your sports kit. It becomes easier to get to the pub rather than the gym. Worst of all, you'll find exercise becoming a bit of a chore. If you keep doing the same routine every time you exercise you'll inevitably reach a stage when you feel stuck in the mud.

This is where you need to switch on! It's not as bad as it seems – everyone hits these plateaus, and as you gain more experience you'll know what to do. First, assess whether there are other reasons for your tiredness and lack of enthusiasm. Don't panic. Accept it. Make sure you're still just wooing it in; take a break, lower the intensity, or raise the intensity and work for less time. One common reason for the plateau is that inexperienced, out-of-condition exercisers see positive changes within the first few weeks, but the improvements don't keep happening this quickly. Eventually your body will grow more tolerant to exercise and you have to raise the intensity or change what you are doing. If your body is growing tolerant to your routine in the same week that other pressures are getting you down, it can just be too much. Be on the lookout for the plateau, add a bit of variety and don't get despondent! The results will keep coming if you are persistent and consistent.

'Today I won Wimbledon'

I heard a story about the tennis champion Martina Navratilova. For a whole year before Wimbledon she wrote in her diary, 'Today I won Wimbledon'. After writing it down every day she convinced herself and reinforced her goal on a daily basis. By the time the competition started I reckon she had won. How much time does it take to write a few words: 'Today I ran 6 miles', 'Today I got into my favourite jeans', 'Today I swam a mile'. As you write your goal down every day, watch over a short space of time how you become focused, how things snowball in a positive way and you realise you will achieve your goal.

Think how you will react when doubts creep in. Some will knock you back, and some people will give up forever. Do you want to be one of those people? It's worth considering these challenges before you start. Have faith, continue to keep everything simple, stay frosty and woo exercise into your life. The consistency needs to come before you get a whiff of success. You have to deal with it and slog it out. There's no other way I'm afraid. But if you are prepared for these setbacks you'll be better equipped to deal with each one effectively. Keep everything simple. Be consistent, enjoy it, exercise little and often. Have faith in yourself.

'Success is on the other side of frustration.'

Anthony Robbins

Chapter 9

Myths, mistakes, old wives tales and 'my mate up the pub said...'

The title of this chapter says it all, and it's a lot easier and more efficient to learn from other people's mistakes. You'll achieve your objectives a lot quicker and enjoy exercise more. So, here are some of the myths about exercise...

Everyone in the gym knows what they're doing

It can be intimidating to enter the atmosphere of a gym or health club – they're not always the most welcoming places, especially for a newcomer. One thing I can guarantee, though, is that most punters are just cracking on with their own personal challenges and battles, so don't let them put you off. As for knowing what they're doing, the truth is most people could make their exercise regime more effective, but if they are exercising in a *safe*, *enjoyable* way and are *consistent* then that's good enough! Nothing lasts forever, and your initial unease will soon wear off.

I haven't exercised for a whole week and I've lost all my fitness gains

First of all you need to figure out why you haven't exercised. It's not the end of the world, but perhaps you've just been trying to do too much or life has got in the way and you feel demotivated. Understanding the reasons will help you prepare for the next time it happens.

The positive side is that you haven't exercised for a week and still want to get back into your routine. If you've only been exercising for a few days before having a week off, it's not a great start. However, if you've exercised *consistently* for a number of weeks prior to your break then don't sweat the time off. The longer your routine has been consistent, the lower the chances that you're really back to square one. Regardless of where you are on your fitness campaign, it's more important to assess why you stopped in the first place. Next – get over it! Forget it and get exercising again. Enjoy it, ease back into the first couple of sessions and your fitness levels will quickly return. You're further down the line than you think, and you've just overcome another challenge, which can only be a positive thing.

A good bout of hard exercise will sweat out last night's beer

Stop! Your body will be working hard to recover from the toxins and effects of alcohol. You'll be dehydrated and feel tired from ineffective sleep. You won't get much out of a visit to the gym, so stick to a walk in the fresh air. Wait until you've recovered and can have a more worthwhile bout of exercise. If you do decide to exercise then make sure you're rehydrated before you begin, and lower the intensity of your normal routine. Keep it short with plenty of rest, and drink water before, during and after your workout. I guarantee the first bout of exercise after a big party won't be particularly fun, so accept it.

The best thing to do if you have a cold is to sweat it out in the gym and finish with a sauna

You won't sweat anything out, all you'll do is spread your germs around the gym and sauna. You are ill for a reason and your body is telling you to stop. Listen to it. Your immune system will be low, your body will be working hard to get you back to good health, so help it out.

I once read an article by a doctor for the Great Britain Olympic team. She discussed the differences of being ill from the neck up and the neck down. If your symptoms are neck down, i.e. aching limbs, stomach pains, then you definitely shouldn't exercise. If your symptoms are neck up, i.e. headache, runny nose, then exercise won't do you any harm, but make sure it's very light, easy and short. You won't sweat out a cold. If you exercise too much when you're unwell you'll make yourself worse, so you need to be sensible, listen to the signs from your body and seek professional medical advice if you're unsure.

Maria

Maria had been a regular exerciser for a number of years and exercised four or five times a week. She worked full time and exercised three mornings a week and ran with a running club two evenings a week. Maria stopped exercising when she found out she was pregnant simply because she felt constantly tired. After her son was born the only exercise she was able to do was walking the pram, until it became easier to find a routine. When the baby was about six months old Maria began to exercise two or three times a week. This would consist of 20-minute bouts of walking and jogging. The next stage was to design a programme around being a full-time mother and housewife. It was not practical to leave her son, so a home programme with minimum equipment was needed. We aimed to do short bouts of exercise throughout the day that wouldn't interfere with the baby's routine. Self-discipline and motivation was required with simplicity and *consistency* the key. We planned the following exercises, to be done throughout the day:

- Press-ups   2 x 8–12 reps
- Hip raises   2 x 8–12 reps
- Plank   2 x 15 seconds
- Lunges   2 x 12 reps
- Bent over row   2 x 12 reps
- Bench dips   2 x 8 reps

Maria had to work her way through these exercises four days a week. Sometimes it was not practical to do them all in one go, so she did them at random times throughout the day depending on when the baby slept and how energetic she felt! Some days she had completed them by late morning and at other times would do them in the evening. It didn't matter – the aim was just to get her body used to doing exercise again. The exercises required the minimum amount of equipment and worked all major muscle groups. They were designed to be just enough to keep her motivated without feeling she had to start again from scratch. Maria had previously exercised a lot so her body soon adapted to exercise again. It was the simplest and most practical routine but the *consistency* enabled her body to get used to exercise again.

You should always stretch before you exercise

It's okay to stretch before you exercise but it will be more beneficial to stretch on completion. Whatever you do, make sure your muscles are warm before you stretch. Your joints should be moving easily and your inner body should feel warm. Don't just start stretching, get moving first. During exercise your muscles are contracting and shortening, so spend some time easing down at the end of your routine to lower your heart rate and keep warm. Stretching and relaxing at the end is a good way to wind down and be happy that you have exercised. Don't rush it.

I have a bad back so I can't exercise

If you are concerned about the effects of exercise on your back then it goes without saying you need professional advice from a doctor or physiotherapist before you start. Establish what exercises may cause problems for your back and avoid them. Once you have the all-clear then exercise can improve your mobility and the strength of your back and core muscles, but make sure you listen to your body.

Loads of stomach exercises will give you a flat tummy

I'm afraid not. If you want to improve your waist, or even go as far as getting a six-pack, it's all down to *consistent* exercise and what you eat. Just concentrating on sit-ups will be wasted energy. Exercise on a regular basis will work – aerobic exercise with big movements to raise your heart rate and sustain it. Strength work that involves big compound exercises (lots of muscle groups) and core work will also help. If you want a flat tummy, *move more, eat less*.

Now I'm exercising a lot more I can eat what I want

Don't kid yourself. Why put in all that hard work and then feed yourself with empty food? To burn up a single pound of fat (approx 3,500 calories) it will take a lot of hard graft. That's seven hours of exercise burning 500 calories per hour. Enjoy treats, by all means, but prioritise your food needs and keep your body topped up with good fuel.

You've probably come across a few of the myths in this chapter. It all comes back to the basic principles of safe, enjoyable and consistent exercise if you want to succeed.

Chapter 10

Common mistakes

This chapter is the closest you'll ever get to a shortcut to fitness. It will make you a lot more efficient when exercising. After all, you'd be very disappointed if you spent hours exercising only to discover you could have been more effective. If you're going to waste time, do it somewhere else. Here's how to work efficiently and effectively when exercising.

Preparing for an outdoor run on a treadmill
Running on a treadmill is beneficial and can build your confidence before attempting to run outside. It should at least be warm and dry inside your gym! It won't be dark, there are no little dogs to nibble your ankles and a hot shower is only an emergency stop button away. The treadmill will also help your pace judgement, as most have screens that tell you how fast you're running and offer a different choice of workouts. If you're really lucky there'll even be a TV screen to distract you! The running machine is a good way to help improve your fitness.

However, once you've built up your stamina and confidence you can't beat a good old-fashioned run in the fresh air to strengthen your immune system. It's a lot more challenging running outside. The ground is not moving for you, hills appear when they shouldn't, rain, snow and howling winds will challenge your motivation. But it's free, no one can stop you, skin is waterproof, you won't have to queue, there's no recycled air from fellow gym users, and you get to wave at other crazy joggers as well. The other great thing is that you can do it anywhere – just pack your kit when you go away on business, on holiday or for a visit to the mother-in-law. I often visited foreign ports when I was in the Navy. I'd go running with the lads and saw sights I would never have seen if I'd been in a taxi (or the local police cell)…

So, if you've entered the local 30-mile mud run for charity after a drunken bet, you need to get outside! Don't cancel your gym membership, but gradually start to swap an indoor run for an outdoor run once a week. Make the transition slowly to let your body adapt. Your pace judgement will take a bit of getting used to. If you're used to running for 30 minutes at the gym, swap it for a 20-minute run and walk outside. Don't run too fast in the first mile – remember, you still have to get back. Take a training buddy with you for support, but make sure you choose someone who will be happy to run *with* you and not over you!

Becoming a runner

I'm a great believer in doing exercise that you enjoy because you'll never make it part of your life forever if you don't feel good or don't improve. Many people who come to me after a break from exercise tell me that they don't like running, they don't want to run, that they can't run. Of course, there are plenty of other ways of exercising if you're a bit out of condition or carrying too much weight. However, a lot of people I meet would like to incorporate some running into their programme but are wary of starting. Not many of us want to run outside for the first time, being exposed to the elements and feeling we are on show to the whole world. It's not very encouraging either, jogging on a treadmill when a Paula Radcliffe lookalike jumps on next to you! And a few bad memories of cross-country running at school will be the nail in the coffin.

If you feel that you honestly can't run or don't want to then that's fine, but don't dismiss it forever. If you're exercising regularly and getting good results, then keep doing that. However, if you are in good health there are a lot of benefits to adding some running to your routine, and I have plenty of tips to encourage you. For a start, you only need a decent pair of trainers and you can do it absolutely anywhere – you'll never have an excuse not to exercise when you are away on business or holiday!

Once you've decided that you really want to start running, think about it positively, stamp out any negative thoughts or memories now.

Don't start until you've given yourself a good reason to – and a goal. You don't have to sign up for a marathon, just find an achievable goal to keep you focused and motivated. Make sure that you have successfully wooed in your exercise and that it has become a part of your routine. At this stage it's beneficial to have experienced challenging weeks. Make sure you've worked through the exercises from the Six for Life routine (see page 78) for at least 4–6 weeks before you start to run. This should build your strength and prepare you to run.

If you're nervous about running then don't drop your usual routine completely. Incorporate a little running depending on your fitness levels. Remember – it's better to walk away feeling you could have done more rather than doing too much. Try swapping 10 minutes on the bike for a 10-minute walk and run if you're in the gym just to get a feel for it. Dave's 'Simple but Special' on page 99 is an excellent way to start running, and there are some other ideas in that section, too.

You don't have to run to get fit, but it's a very practical and simple way of getting results. Anyone can do it, as long as they are prepared physically and mentally, have set achievable goals, can maintain their sense of humour and have some self-belief. Trust me you'll be surprised at how much you can do.

Dealing with your least-favourite exercise

Everyone has an exercise that they dread. This is normal – they can't all be your favourite, after all. There are always alternative exercises to target each body part, so if there is a particular exercise you really despise, the simple answer is don't do it! However, when I scratch below the surface I often find that people want to improve at a certain exercise, but just don't feel competent at it. If there's an exercise you don't like, but you know will be beneficial (such as for rehabilitation after an injury) you'll probably leave it to the end of your workout, avoid it or not do it at all. And therein lies the problem. Don't leave it until you're tired and thinking about your shower. Do it at the beginning when you've warmed up and are feeling fresh. You'll soon change how you feel about it. A typical example is someone saying, 'I hate the rowing machine'. I look at their routine and find they do 20 minutes of running, 20 minutes of cycling, then get on the rower but only last five minutes! In this case, either don't row, or swap the order and do five minutes rowing at the beginning. Then keep adding on the minutes on the rower and perhaps lose some time on the bike. This way you'll slowly get stronger on the rowing machine without making your workout longer.

Exercising during time off, and stopping when you are busy

If you find yourself with a long period of free time, make the most of it! Seasonal workers, oil-rig workers, students or teachers may have an opportunity for a regular break of six weeks or more. If you haven't managed to get consistent with exercise prior to your break then some time out could give you an opportunity for that kick-start. But what happens when life goes back to normal? It's possible to go from one extreme to the other – loads of exercise to hardly any – and then end up stopping completely. After all that achievement what will you do when the break is over and you're back to that crazy schedule? During the break will you woo exercise into your life or grab it kicking and screaming? Just make sure you have a thorough plan for when life returns to normal; you may have to woo it in again when the break is over. Just accept that it will be challenging to fit in your exercise when you're back at work or studying, and you may have to ease off the gas. Stay consistent. You've had the potential to achieve a lot during your break, don't let the hard work go to waste.

Dame Kelly Holmes is an inspirational athlete who in the past faced constant setbacks with injuries, but every time she got knocked back became more determined. After all her hard work, determination and pure stubbornness, she won two Olympic gold medals in the space of a few days. When you get a setback, accept it, crack on and *be consistently persistent.*

Maybe you can relate to a few of the examples in this chapter. Make a mental note of them – and reread them if necessary.

Where and how will you get started?

This section will help you decide whether to join a gym or health club, or whether you are going to exercise at home or outside. Once you've made that decision you'll know what type of exercise to do. In the following chapters are some tips for exercising on your own, in small or large groups.

Chapter 11

Where will you exercise?

By now you should be feeling positive about your new exercise-for-life regime. You should be practising your visualisation and positive thinking to enhance your confidence and self-belief. But before you run off and invest a load of money in gym membership, have a think.

Joining a gym or health club

You don't have to join a gym or a health club to exercise; there's plenty of opportunity to exercise outdoors or at home. The problem with trying to get fit at home is that the fridge, TV controls, kids and phone are never far away. There are many distractions and it's not always a conducive environment to get motivated if you lack self-discipline.

The advantage of the gym is that once you're there amongst the equipment and like-minded people there are few distractions and it can be easier to exercise. It's probably one of the few places where you can manage some time for yourself. There should be expert advice readily available, as well as different classes and good equipment to suit all ages and abilities to aid self-motivation.

If you're thinking about joining a fitness centre there are plenty of things to take into account before signing up. No matter how difficult it is, make sure you start exercising before you join, even if it's just walking or running outside with some 'Six For Life' exercises thrown in at home. If you can do it that way round and keep it up, you'll be in a better place physically and mentally before committing yourself and spending any money. If you can't do that then consider a 'pay as you go' gym so you can get a feel for what you prefer.

The influx of new members to most fitness centres takes a massive bump in January. Things settle back to normal at the end of February before a fresh influx joins in preparation for getting into their summer clothes. Whatever time of the year you intend to join – and for whatever reason – seriously consider your weekly routine. It's all well and good going somewhere with cutting-edge equipment and lots of punters wearing the latest sports kit, but honestly a gym is a gym! It's also easy to fall into the trap of believing once you've joined and committed to the monthly payments you'll definitely go.

If you are adamant you are going to join, make sure you view the premises and facilities at the time you intend to exercise there. The place could have a quiet and relaxed library atmosphere at 10 a.m., but a completely different atmosphere at 5.30 p.m. with blaring club music, testosterone and lipstick everywhere, and fashion victims all hogging the equipment. Whatever floats your boat! Maybe you are a social person and would prefer a club with sociable staff and members. That won't work for you if you prefer to exercise alone in a spacious environment.

Everyone has their own tastes and preferences so it's up to you, but location will probably be the deciding factor. Give some thought to when you are going to visit the gym. Will it be before work, in your lunch break or immediately after work? It might make sense to join somewhere close to work, which is okay if you don't plan to exercise at the gym on your days off or at weekends. If you join somewhere closer to home, will you feel like going back out to the gym after sitting in rush-hour traffic on the way home? Ideally you should be able to mix up your exercise venues, some in the gym and some outside in the fresh air. This will give you more flexibility, a change of scenery – and fewer reasons not to do it! Some people like to go for the social scene and join the same club as friends or work colleagues, but make sure you pick the place that suits your routine. If you and your friends will encourage each other that's great, but if their motivation slips away will you go it alone?

Fitness classes
A major advantage of joining a gym or health club is that most offer organised classes that can add variety to your exercise routine. There are plenty of advantages to joining a class: you won't have to decide what

to do, the instructor will make the decision for you; it's generally harder to finish early in a group, unlike when you train alone; and a little bit of competition could make you work harder. The atmosphere of a good class can encourage you to keep going and if the music suits your taste, then even better!

The disadvantage of classes is that you have to work your routine around the timetable, and popular classes at the most convenient times can cramp your personal space. The classes are designed for groups of all different abilities, so it may be too challenging or too easy. The competition element can sometimes get a bit much for some people in a cramped studio. Banging club music and testosterone climbing up the walls is not everyone's cup of tea.

If you're just starting out then try a variety of classes to see what works for you. If you participate in classes make sure you exercise on your own as well. This means that if your favourite instructor or class is permanently cancelled you won't feel at a loss. It will also prevent you relying solely on classes to get motivated – never pass responsibility for your motivation to someone else. If you have the balance right, then your personal sessions should enhance your class abilities and vice versa.

Pick a class that challenges you in a positive way and makes you feel revitalised and encouraged. It can be a bit intimidating walking into a class where everyone seems to know each other, and they all know the moves and exercises. Just be patient, nothing lasts forever, and once you've done a few classes taking part will come more easily. Just walk in like you own the place!

Special offers

Special offers are a good way of enticing new members to join health clubs and gyms. Examples such as 3–15 day temporary memberships are common. It's great if you're in two minds about joining somewhere and want to get a feel for the place to see if it will suit you. This could give you that little nudge to get your new fitness campaign off to a special start. If it happens to be over a two-week period there's a good chance you'll see positive changes after living a sedentary lifestyle for a few years!

If you've upped the exercise intensity for your two-week membership, ask yourself if you'll keep it up. It will be easy to get motivated if you have a short-term membership, you'll want to get your money's worth for the two weeks, and will probably end up using all the equipment, participate in all the classes and make the most of the free shower gel!

Think about the principles at the beginning of the book, though. You have to woo exercise into your life. Take your time and ensure you give it plenty of thought. Be a little cheeky and ask for another two-week membership to ensure you keep up the routine! You will definitely have a more realistic insight after four weeks.

Ask yourself why you are joining the gym and what you want from it. It has to be practical and easy to get to regardless of the cutting-edge equipment and facilities. This exercise regime is going to last, so you want to feel comfortable and look forward to going for some time out. It will have to enhance your exercise lifestyle and give you the minimum reasons not to go!

Chapter 12

Warming up, warming down and stretching

What shall we do with a drunken sailor?

One of my responsibilities onboard ship was to act as quartermaster when we were in dock. I could probably write another book about the happenings and sights I witnessed of sailors returning from a 'run ashore'. It was 1.30 a.m., the ship was alongside in Plymouth and I was just about to go off watch. An old and bold able seaman returned after a mammoth 12-hour endurance exercise in the local drinking holes. He had his Chinese takeaway in both hands, but decided to convince the gangway staff he could easily lift the weight-training bar left in the ship's hanger before he went to get his head down. Well you can never win an argument with a drunken sailor and 10 minutes later we were packing him in an ambulance after he had lifted the weight, fallen backwards and dropped it on his head!

It's not safe to jump off the settee and run around the block like a Tasmanian devil. It's definitely not healthy to dive back through the front door and instantly slump on the settee again. You need to prepare your body to exercise, give it a bit of a warning. When you suddenly have to run for a bus and then stop, you always feel unfit. It's not always a true reflection of your fitness levels, because your heart rate has just overcompensated to get you to react quickly to catch the bus, and your body doesn't have time to prepare. The same goes for normal exercise. It's important, safe, rewarding and effective to make the transition from inactivity to activity and back. Your body will always give you a running commentary and feedback, especially pre- and post-exercise, so just listen to it.

Warming up – before exercise

This is where you prepare your body for the activity. The warm-up will lessen the chance of injury and let your body know you are about to exercise, so you'll be better prepared both physically and mentally. You're making the transition from sitting down to being active. Whatever you're expecting to do in your workout, do it in your warm-up but with a lighter intensity, a smaller range of movement and build on it. It will make sense to wear warm clothes at this time to help increase your body temperature. Start with light aerobic exercise such as walking or light jogging and gradually move on to bigger, whole-body movements. This will mobilise your joints, raise your heart rate and get your blood flowing. Spend between three and five minutes warming up and raising your heart rate. Make it specific. If you're swimming do some light pool exercises, easy swimming and build up from there; if you're going for a run, include a light run in your warm-up. If you're doing circuits and bodyweight exercises then carry out a few of the forthcoming exercises in a light and slow manner after raising your body temperature. At the end of the warm-up your joints should move more easily and you should be better prepared – mentally and physically – and breathing more deeply. You can then make a natural transition into your planned workout.

Easing down – after exercise

The best bit! This is to slow down your heart rate gradually and safely, and to switch from being active to resting. Basically, it's the opposite of your warm-up. If you think like that you won't go far wrong. Keep it simple, just ease off the gas, bring your heart rate down slowly and keep the blood flowing. It depends on what exercise you've done, but like in the warm-up, keep it specific and mirror what you have done but on a lighter scale. This will keep your heart pumping and the blood flowing around the muscles you have just used. Imagine it just slowly flushing through your muscles rather than suddenly stopping and therefore building tension. I know if I've had a tough time on a rowing machine I want to get off and launch it out the window. My natural instinct is to get far away from the thing (they're not designed for people with short legs!). If I do that I'll suffer the next day. Don't make the same mistake;

stay with the kit for a few minutes and let your body catch up. If you've just completed a run, then a light jog or walk, or alternating between both for 3–5 minutes will probably be enough before you stretch. But relax and enjoy it, you should be pleased with yourself.

Stretching – after exercise

Flexibility is the most neglected component of exercise, and lack of flexibility means you have to work harder when exercising and therefore need more energy to perform. Lack of flexibility can cause inefficient technique and poor performance. If your flexibility is improved to increase your range of movement then you'll perform more effectively and reduce the chance of injury. It will be detrimental if you don't work to increase or maintain your flexibility.

Watching some people stretching is like watching WWF wrestling on the TV! I make the same noise a car mechanic makes as he looks under the bonnet and sucks his teeth. Watching inexperienced exercisers rolling around a mat trying to remove legs from hips doesn't make me happy in my work. Stretching should be relaxed, enjoyable and free from pain. Carry out your stretches on completion of your ease-down. Make sure you stay warm, put on another layer of clothing to maintain body heat, and hold the stretches for 20–40 seconds. Do two sets on each stretch. Always stretch the muscles around the hips, hamstrings and back.

You should be physically and mentally relaxed when stretching. Don't get competitive and force your muscles to lengthen. Don't let your mind wander. Stay in tune with your body and move around until the position feels right for you. Aim to feel a mild increase in muscle tension in the central part of the muscle and not the joints. This should be a comfortable sensation of lengthening – there should be no pain. When you feel light tension just stay there for a few seconds, relax your breathing and your muscles should relax a little. Then you can move your body to increase the stretch and feel a mild tension again. Repeat this action as your muscles start to relax. Stay comfortable and enjoy it, feel your body winding down.

Stretch all your major muscle groups and look at developing your flexibility. This will also help you recover more quickly, develop your range of movement, keep you mobile and help you feel refreshed. This is your reward, take your time.

Stretches

Hamstring (back of the thigh)
Kneel down with one knee on the floor and your hips facing forward. Extend the other leg out in front of you with the toe up. Stay tall from the hips, chest out and lean forward slightly. Extend your spine by slightly pushing your behind away.

Hip (hip joint) flexor
Kneel down and place one foot flat in front of you, keeping the knee over the ankle. Place the other leg behind you, with the knee on the floor and the leg and foot extended behind. Keep your hips facing forward and your upper body tall. You should feel a stretch in the front hip of the leg extended behind you.

Quadriceps (front of the thigh)
Lie on your left side supported by your left elbow underneath your shoulder. Keep your knees together and bend your right knee, hold your right foot at the laces with your right hand. Keep your right shoulder, hip and knee in line. Push your right foot into your right hand and gently pull to stretch the upper part of your thigh. Roll over and do the same on the opposite side. If you struggle and are unable to reach your foot, use a towel to wrap around your foot and gently stretch. The same stretch can be done standing with anything sturdy to support you.

Calves (back of lower leg)
Lean into a solid wall and support your body weight with your arms. Place one leg in front of the other with the rear leg straight behind and your toes and hips facing forward. Keep your hips forward and your back flat. Slowly lower the heel of your rear leg until you feel the stretch in the lower leg.

Chest
Stand close to a wall with your arms stretched above your head and your

palms on the wall. Step back slightly and look down through your arms and shoulders to feel a slight stretch in upper chest and arms.

Upper back and shoulders

Stand tall and straighten your right arm across your chest. Lift your chin over your shoulder and look to the right. Hold your right elbow with your left hand and gently pull to increase the stretch. Change over and stretch other side.

Triceps (back of the arms)

Stand tall and put your right hand over the back of your head as if trying to scratch your back. With your left hand hold your right elbow and gently pull behind your head. Change and stretch the other arm.

The warm-up is aimed at preparing you both mentally and physically to start exercising while using the minimum amount of energy. Don't tire yourself out during this phase, look at it as a transition from sitting down to exercising. The ease-down is the same but the other way round, going from exercising to sitting down. Make sure it is a progressive and gradual change in both cases. Listen to your body's feedback, don't overstretch and get competitive.

Chapter 13

You've got your ticket, now get on the bus

'You've got your ticket, but you ain't on the bus yet'
To be selected for Physical Trainers course in the Royal Navy you first have to pass a three-day aptitude test at HMS *Temeraire* in Portsmouth. Luckily for me I attended my aptitude test in December 1985, before anyone at the Royal Navy School of Physical Training had heard of 'investors in people', 'political correctness', 'health and safety' and the Human Rights Act! I had just returned from six months at sea in sunny climes and found myself in the snow, swimming in the open sea at 5 a.m. What a laugh!

I somehow managed to scrape through the three days, and was hoping to start my full course in June 1986. You would have thought I was Superman the way I walked back onboard my ship. I was soon brought down to earth when a wise PT instructor gave me a look and said, 'You've got your ticket, but you ain't on the bus yet.' In other words, 'Don't get cocky sailor, you've got some work to do!'

My PT instructor was right, and that's how you should be thinking before you throw yourself in. You should be well prepared now, so you've already got your ticket. Trouble is, this bus often stops whenever it wants, so don't get off at the wrong stop!

Exercises to get you started and last for life
Every personal trainer, fitness coach and strength conditioner will have a view on the best type of exercise. There's information everywhere on what is most effective, how to achieve amazing results without even raising your heart rate, routines that can make you a better lover, get a

six-pack by Friday or be able to run a marathon! In truth, it all comes down to a few things that we've already covered: *consistent, safe* and *enjoyable* exercise.

Whatever you think is the best for you, I guarantee the 'Six for Life' exercises will work like magic with a well-balanced lifestyle. They are a compact group of exercises that will get you to move more, working all your major muscles and improving your strength and stamina. You'll never regret doing these exercises, whether you're just starting exercise or have always done it. The idea is to learn and practise each exercise so you get a feel for each of them. Don't quickly read through the explanations and then do them every day at the gym. They should be carried out alongside other forms of exercise, such as walking, running or cycling. Knowing how to do them will give you variation, confidence and the opportunity to exercise anywhere and at any time.

So this is it, plenty of focusing on your goals, visualisation and positive thinking is coming to fruition, and you can't wait to get on that bus and get started. But before we start there are a couple of final preps to square away:

- Check any sports kit to ensure all price tags have been removed
- Rub your new trainers with a bit of mud and grit
- Empty old chocolate wrappers and crisp packets out of your sports bag.

Done? We're good to go.

'Six for Life' (6FL) exercises

The following are the six exercises anyone and everyone needs to do. If you want to get fit for life, change how you look or feel, then the 6FLs will work. This is your foundation, and if you practise these six exercises your house will be strong and withstand all weathers. By that I mean these exercises will stand you in good stead forever. They are simple and effective, but each one can be adapted to make them less intensive or more challenging to suit different fitness levels and abilities. When you see improvements they can be slightly changed so you can progressively make them more challenging. You could do them at home in your front room, in your garage, on holiday, in the garden, or do them at the local gym. If you start getting the bug, you could even do them in your hotel room while away on business!

You may have tried some of these exercises before, or at least seen them done. The 6FL exercises do what they say on the tin: six exercises that work all your major muscle groups, using a minimum of equipment and which, once mastered, will prove to be a good long-term investment. I guarantee that any athlete, sportsperson and serious trainer will be doing versions of the 6FLs, and benefiting from them.

To get started, work your way through 2–3 sets of each exercise and do 8–20 reps (repetitions) of each one depending on your fitness levels and ability. Do the 6FLs at least twice a week and no more than three times a week. As you do them, always think '*core blimey*'! In other words, get your stomach and back muscles tuned in, engaged and working. The numbers and aims are not set in stone as you'll quickly improve. Spend the first few times getting a feel for them and find an intensity that is challenging but not exhausting. After you've done them twice a week for three weeks you should start to feel improvements in your technique, strength and stamina. There are more detailed training routines in the exercise programmes further on in the book.

Note:

Repetitions, or reps, are the number of times an exercise is performed without rest. Sets is a group of repetitions. For example, three sets of 15 repetitions will be written as 3 x 15.

'If in doubt – drag it out!'

Top tip! Do the exercises *slowly*. It'll take discipline but you'll get far better results by getting into good habits. Doing these exercises quickly will make them shorter, easier and less effective. Slower movements will be more *effective*.

1. Press-ups

Okay, it's an old fashioned exercise that most people know – and often for the wrong reasons. If you've been in the military or had an old-style PE teacher then you probably think of this as a punishment exercise, so the poor old press-up gets some bad press. Forget all those negative thoughts. There are loads of simple ways of making this exercise more enjoyable and comfortable. It works major upper-body muscles, i.e. chest, shoulders, back of your arms and abdominals. It's a classic exercise, it's practical, you only need your own body weight, it's functional, simple to do and gets results. So come on – have a go!

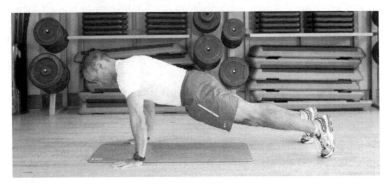

Place your toes and hands on the floor and face the ground. Keep your hands slightly more than a shoulder-width apart, and your body at such an angle that your spine is as flat as naturally possible. Pull your belly button into your spine (suck your tummy in), bend at the elbows and lower your upper body to the floor slowly (3–4 seconds). Your nose and hands should form the three points of a triangle. Stop when you're a few centimetres from the floor, hold for one second and push your

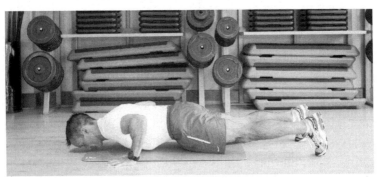

body back up dynamically (2 seconds). To make it easier place your knees on the floor.

2. Plank

This is what I call a 'bus-stop' exercise. You can do it anywhere! Okay, doing it while waiting for a bus is a bit extreme, but you get my drift. Do this one when you're waiting for the kettle to boil, while the adverts are on at home, in the office or in the gym. It's simple and effective, and can be easy or as challenging as you want.

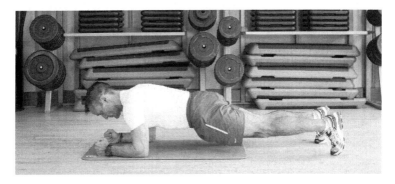

Lie on the floor only supported by your forearms and toes. Look down, pull in your stomach, engage your lower abs, back flat and hips and neck aligned with your spine. Keep that position for anywhere between 20 seconds and one minute. To make it easier, balance on your knees rather than your toes. The next progression is to do the same but rest your forearms on a Swiss ball.

3. Squats

You probably do this exercise every day. It's the same as standing up from your office chair, or slowly sitting back down without using your arms for support. It's a great functional exercise, practical, simple and very effective. It works your major leg muscles and core muscles, it can be aerobically challenging and it forces your whole body to get stronger. There are plenty of different versions of this exercise, and it will prepare you well for your fitness campaign for life. If you choose only one exercise to do for life, this is the one!

Sit on a sturdy bench or chair with the backs of your legs parallel to the floor when you are sitting down. Feet should be a shoulder width apart. Push with your weight through the heels and stand up; press

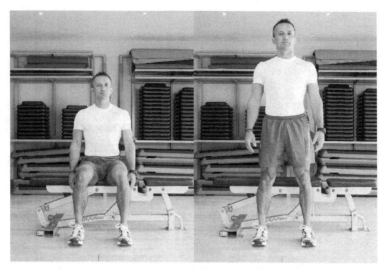

your hips forward. Keep your upper body still, and your back naturally flat with as little movement as possible in your upper body, i.e. stay tall from the hips. When you stand up, don't lock your knees. Slowly lower yourself back down to the bench and repeat. As you get stronger, try to prevent your whole body weight going through your bottom as you sit on the bench, just slightly touch the bench with your behind, hold for a second and stand up again.

4. Bent-over row

Out of all the 6FLs this is probably the most difficult to master, so expect it to take a while and be patient. When you try the previous exercises, you can instantly feel the muscles working. With the bent-over row it takes a bit of time. It just doesn't feel right for some people to begin with, but persevere. The muscles we are trying to target are your lower- and mid-back, stomach and front of your arms. For a start you can't see the muscles in your back, and they can be a little less receptive to your brain's requests. Try to concentrate on pinching your shoulder blades together, and visualise your back muscles working. Most of us need to strengthen our back because of our sedentary lifestyles. It's great for posture and feel-good factor once mastered. Stick this one out – it's a fabulous exercise.

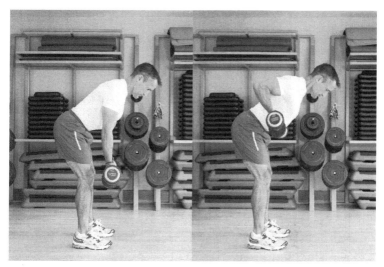

Stand tall, with your feet a shoulder-width apart. Face forward and then lean forward from the hips to about 30 degrees. Keep your stomach tight ('core blimey') and your back flat. Hold a barbell, weights or resistance with your palms up and then pull into your sternum. Think about your posture all the time, elbows close to your body, shoulders back and down towards your hips. Imagine there's a pen between your shoulder blades to grip throughout the movement. Then lower the weight while keeping your shoulders back and your spine flat. Repeat.

Note: The amount of weight you should lift will vary from person to person. The best advice is to lift something that feels light at first. As you do more repetitions it will become more challenging. Light weights and lots of reps (two lots of 15–20 reps) done slowly will build your endurance, confidence and help you get a feel for it. Make sure your form stays the same throughout the exercise.

5. Crunch and push

Forget those old-fashioned sit-ups. This exercise will target your stomach muscles. Imagine your stomach following the initial movement of opening a sardine tin.

Lie on your back with your feet flat on the floor, knees bent with your lower back pushed into the mat. Extend your arms above your

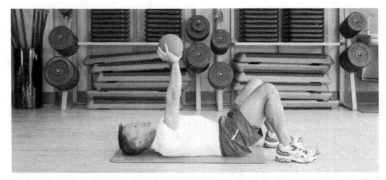

chest. Slowly raise your shoulder blades off of the floor until you feel your stomach muscles tense; keep your arms extended. Look up at the ceiling. Lower your shoulder blades but keep your stomach muscles engaged. Make sure you do not use any momentum, and keep the movement and speed controlled. Keep looking up to keep your back flat. To make this more challenging you can hold something in your hands such as a bag of sugar or a medicine ball.

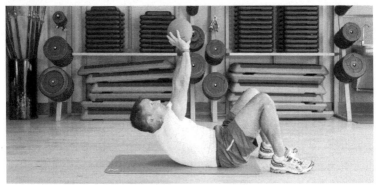

6. Hip raises

This exercise will target the back of your legs, buttocks and core. These muscle groups are often neglected, and it's important to keep them active to encourage a strong lower back and core. This is a simple exercise needing only your own body weight and a bench or chair. Like the others, it can be made more challenging and intensive to suit individual needs.

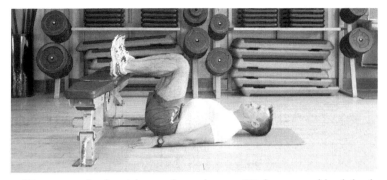

Lie on your back, with your knees bent at 90 degrees and both heels on the bench or chair. Keep your shoulders and upper back on the floor and gently raise your hips so your stomach, hips and upper thighs make a straight line. Keep your stomach and back tight and then slowly lower. To make it more challenging do more repetitions, or do it with only one leg. When you feel stronger, start using a Swiss ball instead of the bench.

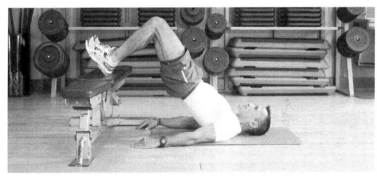

You'll find some of these exercises easy and others more challenging, but don't worry – it will all get easier as you progress. All six of them will give you an excellent base from which to further your goals. Even if you do plenty of exercise you'll still benefit from *consistently* doing the 6FLs.

Chapter 14

The easiest and most direct route to your goal

It's a big achievement to exercise on a regular basis and discover you've successfully wooed exercise into your life, but it's important to keep having a word with yourself just to reassess where you are on the exercise path, and whether or not you are still feeling positive. You should be confident and notice that everything is in balance. Exercise shouldn't be preventing you from the achievements of daily life, and vice versa. Make sure exercise is a long-term commitment and accept that you'll always be learning new things. Don't try and move on too quickly. If you're happy, you can begin to focus on the intensity of your exercise, and perhaps narrow your sights to a more definitive target.

Get in, get on with it and get out!

The flight deck of a ship is the best place in the world to do exercise with a group of like-minded people. You can't beat exercising at sea – no land in sight, cool sea breeze, sun coming up or going down depending on what time 'flight deck circuits' are happening. There's always good support, as many of the ship's company will be keen to get out of uniform and have a good sweat session 'up top'. It's never formal and with up to three sessions a day on a six-month deployment, it stretches the ship's PT instructor to use his imagination.

So, after a few months away the lads and lasses are getting in good shape and working up the beer credits for the foreign runs ashore. The last flight-deck circuit before a few nights alongside is always special, particularly if you're going somewhere exotic with good night life! The longer you're at sea the fitter the ship's company becomes. It's part of a daily routine for many onboard and gives them a break from the normal working day. I began to realise that the more the group exercised the quicker their bodies were adapting to the rigorous challenges I set. Each individual would become a lot more aware of his/her own limitations, and because of that, less time could be spent warming up and explaining the exercises. The more you exercise, the quicker your body will adapt, and your brain will send more efficient signals to the rest of your body. Everything will start to flow and it will become less of a chore.

The ship's flight deck is a sought-after place, swapping between fitness area, helicopter landing pad, live firing range, barbecue area, church and garage, so sessions sometimes have to be shortened. With a group of familiar and experienced exercisers (you could soon include yourself), 20 or 30 minutes can be enough to get a good session, because you can really raise the tempo and intensity for a short space of time. So 'get in, get on with it and get out!'

Working hard or taking it easy – finding an intensity that works for you

Exercise has to be all about you. Your thoughts, feelings and views may be completely different to someone else's when it comes to exercise, especially your interpretations of working hard! But that's good, it would be very boring if we all had to do the same thing and work the same way to achieve our goals. The problem is we all get sucked into what someone else is doing. We might watch a fly-on-the-wall fitness programme and witness unfit people looking dejected, tired out and less than enthusiastic about their exercise programme. The secret is not to pay attention to what everyone else is trying to do.

I hope by now you have already started an exercise regime and are working towards a *safe, enjoyable* and *consistent* routine. That is far more important than the intensity you feel you need to get positive results. It will take a bit of time to establish your own intensity levels, a bit of 'suck it and see' is the only way! If you've had a break from exercise for a while, start off doing something light. Keep your sessions short and feel like you could do a bit more when you've completed your workout. You'll be more enthusiastic about coming back for another session, and that's far more effective than working so intensively that you feel drained and ache for days afterwards. *So be patient!*

The advantage of being *consistent* is that you'll feel your way into your exercise programme, and as you do that you'll find an intensity that you can sustain for a practical time. If you're trying new types of exercise then inevitably you'll get new aches as your body uses previously un-worked muscles. Sometimes that can feel rewarding, though – you feel like your body is changing and that you have achieved something. If you are permanently tired and drained then you're probably overdoing it. If it's really easy, start increasing the intensity of your exercise by resting less, moving faster or adding a few minutes on to your workout. But make sure you increase using *one* of those principles, not all three at once!

The best advice, the best feedback, the most qualified debrief will come from your own body. Just be patient and listen to what it's telling you every day, accept that you are going to exercise forever so there's no need to go rushing in. You'll soon gain in experience and discover what you can do. Start slowly, build gradually, be patient, *think and stay positive*!

A simple enjoyable routine done consistently is the most effective training programme ever.

3 Gs – get in, get on with it and get out!

By now you should have established an exercise routine that suits your life and your daily regime. You'll start to build on your first few weeks and will probably have a few mishaps – a few days when you just can't manage it – but you'll start to get a better feel for exercise. If you were out of condition at first, you'll see positive changes within the first few weeks and that will steadily improve as you stay *consistent*. Your pace judgement will get better, you'll have a better understanding of what your body is capable of, and you'll be clearer about your physical limits. If you've always exercised you'll already have a good idea about these limits, but if you're just starting it could take a month or so. If you follow all the guidelines and stick to them thoroughly, you'll see plenty of improvements.

When all this comes together you'll feel a lot more confident about exercising. You may not be lucky (or unlucky) enough to have a ship's PTI to keep an eye on you, so make sure you're aware and continually reassess where you are with your goals. Find five minutes a day with no distractions, somewhere comfortable, quiet and where you can be alone. Ask yourself how you feel and how close you are to reaching your short-, mid- or long-term goals. This will keep you focused and encourage you to stay *consistent* and determined. If you've reached this point then it's time to introduce the 3 Gs: 'Get in there, get on with it and get out'.

There are plenty of wonderful places I'd like to waste time: on the beach, in a good restaurant, or just at home in my back garden. I'm sure you have your favourite time-wasting places. Exercise and the gym should not be one of them. Don't waste a single second when you're exercising. Get as much good value as you can out of each minute. Make the most of it, enjoy the moment and be as effective as possible once you have wooed exercise into your life. That doesn't mean you have to work longer and harder – not at all. Even if it's for 10 minutes, get into it and don't be anywhere else! Don't be the kid at the back of the class looking out of the window. Be clear in your mind why you are doing each bout of exercise, even if it's only for a short period. Get in the moment and don't let your mind wander.

'Eyes in the boat!'

It can be dangerous at times going through choppy waters in a Navy inflatable boat. The coxswain is responsible for everyone's safety, and an old Navy statement – 'Eyes in the boat' – just reminds you to focus on what you are doing.

When you exercise, do it with drive and enthusiasm. Watch, listen and feel how your body is reacting to it all, be more aware of your heart rate, your breathing, your inner body temperature, muscular movement and just get into the physicality of it all. It may seem strange at first and take some self-discipline, but it will concentrate your mind and clear your head. When you're done you'll feel physically and mentally refreshed and recharged!

> 'I believe in quality not quantity. You don't see us in the gym for hours on end at Wasps. It's easier to go at 100 per cent for a whole session if it's short.'
>
> Joe Worsley, Wasps, England and British Lions rugby player

Barracuda surf rowing team

Barracuda rowing team consisted of four guys who competed in surf rowing competitions throughout Devon and Cornwall. In 2008 they had been training hard but with no definite routine and programme. They trained *consistently*, sometimes alone or with each other with a 'What shall we do today?' programme – and they finished eighth at the end of the 2008 season. We got together in preparation for the 2009 season and started training in November 2008. I wanted to get them training in a more *consistently* effective way. The previous season they had trained in a quantitative way but not qualitative, i.e. they had been wasting valuable energy.

I was asked to design a programme to get them stronger and faster in the boat, in a way that would work alongside their rowing training and surf-boat drills. They didn't need any motivation, they had already been training *consistently* and were determined to improve. The programme involved big compound (major muscle group) exercises that could be carried out in the gym using a minimum of equipment.

The season started in May 2009 so in November 2008 we concentrated on good technique, muscular and core endurance and general fitness. When they couldn't train together they needed a routine that could be done at home or in their garage. The programme used light weights and high-repetition workouts three times a week, normally Monday, Wednesday and Friday, and was as follows:

- Power cleans   3 x 20 reps
- Bent over row   3 x 20 reps
- Squats   3 x 20 reps
- Dumbbell chest press   3 x 20 reps
- Upright row   3 x 20 reps
- Half jacks   3 x 20 reps
- Plank   3 x 30 secs

The next stage, in January 2009, was to concentrate on pure strength, so we did exactly the same exercises but increased the weights for the first five weight-training exercises and did three sets of eight repetitions. I wanted them to find a weight/resistance that was just achievable but challenging to do eight reps slowly and with good form. This is a very simple and effective way to improve strength after two months of endurance work.

In March 2009 the season was approaching so the next stage was to concentrate on improving their speed and power. We kept the same exercises with three sets of eight repetitions, but slightly decreased the weight/resistance and focused on doing the exercises in a more dynamic way, but with good form.

With the above programme, each crew member's strength and fitness improved dramatically, and this had a positive effect on their motivation and self-belief. The programme was simple, progressive, effective and done in a *consistent* way!

In the league they finished second behind the European champions, and they won the European Championships in Newquay, Cornwall, in September 2009.

Starting at home

The next section will provide plenty of examples of how to organise exercise into your everyday life, and provide numerous opportunities to exercise. It takes a little extra motivation to exercise from home, but you won't look back once you start.

Chapter 15

Exercise routines for non-gym users

This chapter is designed for non-gym members or readers wanting to exercise at home or outdoors. All you need are training shoes, open ground, floor space with a carpet or mat, and a bench or chair.

Making the most of your time

The aim of this chapter is to give you an insight into exercising using your own bodyweight in your home or outdoors without encroaching on your time. It does take a bit more motivation to start exercising at or from home but can save time and money. The sessions are also good for gym users who can't make it to the gym for any reason. You may have to stay at home to look after the kids, or you might be waiting for the new bed to arrive. Chuck in a 15-minute workout before you get sucked into the daytime TV!

However, don't throw yourself into the first exercise programme you see and then set about working your way through them all. Read through the exercise programmes and get a feel for them, choose the one you like the sound of and have a go. You can do them anywhere, on holiday, in prison, at home, on business, on an oil platform or in your garage. Find your favourites but over a period of time try other routines.

Exercising using your own bodyweight is very simple, effective, practical, functional and very, very challenging. There are routines to suit beginners or highly motivated athletes, and they can be adjusted to suit you. It's a way of giving you ideas and showing you practical ways of exercising for life.

Dave's daily dose

This simple exercise routine could give you a gentle push to start exercising. Pick a point in your house that you pass often, such as the bottom of the stairs or kitchen door. For two or three days, every time you pass that point, carry out one of three exercises – knee press-ups, plank or squats. Alternate the exercises as you go on but choose an easy number of repetitions for each, somewhere between six and 12 reps depending on your levels of fitness. At first you might feel a bit daft and at times it may seem rather impractical, but not only will it be entertainment for the other members of your household, you'll also be surprised how quickly you'll improve. Each exercise will only take a few seconds but I guarantee you will be pleasantly surprised at how quickly your body adapts. Just make sure you are warm and your joints are mobilised.

You and three

Pick three exercises that only require your bodyweight and maybe sturdy furniture – step-ups, squats, bench dips or knee press-ups, for example. Choose an upper-body exercise, stomach and a leg exercise that you find challenging. Carry out two sets of 6–20 reps of each, depending on your levels of fitness, three times a day, perhaps once before work, once when you get home and once later in the evening. Warm up properly before you start and stretch on completion. Try it for a few days, but if you keep it up for a week that would be fabulous! This is an effective way to get exercise back into your life – nice and simple and not time-consuming.

Funky 12

If you want to get started after a long break from exercise then this one will work. It's simple, easy and effective. All you have to do is some form of exercise lasting 12 minutes every day, from Monday to Friday. But you always have to do 12 minutes or more continuously. If you decide to do 24 minutes on one day you still have to do 12 minutes the next day. It can be any form of exercise – walking home, gardening, 6FLs, dancing, swimming, skipping… This will add up to one hour a week of exercise. Over a year that's the equivalent of 52 one-hour workouts, or 104 30-minute workouts!

The idea is to make small adjustments to your daily routine to welcome exercise into your life. It will become a habit and the 12 minutes will lead to more. Your body will adapt to it. It's also not such a massive trauma as thinking about other forms of exercise that will take up your day. It allows you a rest from exercise at the weekend; you can exercise then if you want to, but you still have to exercise religiously for 12 minutes every day from Monday to Friday. The only time you don't exercise is when your body tells you not to, i.e. if you are ill or injured.

'Walk the kids to school' workout

If you're struggling to find time to exercise while looking after the kids, doing the housework and going to work, then this is the answer. If your children's school is within walking distance then try this two or three times a week. Once you've dropped the kids off, simply take a different route home – one that adds another 10 or 15 minutes to your journey. You'll already be outdoors so why not spend a few minutes exercising on your way home? As you progress and manage this twice a week you could make it more challenging by finding ways of making the walk longer – or you could even run home.

Try walking the kids to school as you push your bike and then take a bike ride home to add a bit of variety to your workout. This routine will take a bit of discipline and motivation, but it has lots of advantages. For a start, you and your children will benefit from the walk; it will save a journey to the gym; you've done your warm up already by walking your kids; your kids will see you exercising and it could sow the seed for the rest of their lives. It's cheap, simple and practical. As for time, it might take you 10 minutes to walk home the usual way, but by taking a different route and walking hard or jogging for 20 minutes, you've only lost 10 minutes from your day.

Rush-hour workout

Think about how you could make better use of the time spent stuck in rush-hour traffic going to or from work. For example, if you leave for work at 8 a.m. you might spend 45 minutes to an hour travelling just a short distance. If you left anywhere between 20–40 minutes earlier there will probably be a significant drop in travel time due to less traffic.

If that's the case, why not leave earlier and try and exercise when you get to work? If you have shower facilities at work that's perfect. You might even have a gym, a swimming pool or open fields close by.

All you have to do two or three times a week is get out of bed a bit earlier, travel to your workplace earlier and then exercise for 20 minutes. To be honest it's a no-brainer! It might feel a bit strange exercising near work, but just do it and work colleagues will soon get used to it. They may tease you at first but they're probably only jealous! Look at all the advantages you'll gain. For a start, you'll get a better night's sleep as your body clock adjusts to early morning exercise. You'll also avoid wasting time getting stressed in rush-hour traffic, and instead can spend the relaxed journey getting in a good frame of mind for the day. Twenty to 30 minutes of exercise before work will raise your metabolic rate for the morning and get you feeling energised before the day so you'll work more effectively. As you kick down the office door after your shower, make sure you smile and shout 'Good morning!' in a self-righteous way at your sleepy mattress-faced work mates!

I promise you, once you start to do this you'll never look back. You won't believe how good you'll feel the whole day and every day! Once it becomes part of your routine, build on it. Do it every day instead of twice a week. It could be the best decision you ever made in your workplace.

Out back and home

Time for some fresh air. Pick a safe route from your home and walk fast or jog for 15 minutes. Then just turn around, do the same and head for home. Make a mental note of the point you reached before turning around. Do this workout two or three times a week for a few weeks. After a while you'll travel further in the 15 minutes out, and may even run for longer. You'll find it motivating to pass the point you reached on the first attempt, and visually see the distance improve. If you want to challenge yourself more, go for a little longer or pick a route with a few hills.

Sexy cycle

Cycle to work one morning a week. Leave your bike at your workplace and get a lift or the bus home. Two days later, get a lift or the bus in. Cycle home. Over the coming weeks, gradually get used to cycling to and from work. Eventually, you'll be cycling to work every day and never look back.

Harry homers

Twenty-two years in the Royal Navy waiting for transport to get me and the lads back onboard gave me the idea for this routine. I tried it on a client, but only once. Luckily he was mentally stable, quite resilient and had a brilliant sense of humour! I arranged to pick him up and proceeded to drive five miles from his house. I dropped him off and then drove off. I made sure I waited for him at his house and got the kettle on for when he got back.

If your partner picks you up from work every day, once or twice a week greet them in your bright-yellow running kit and jump out of the car a few miles from home to race them back. Once they realise how much fun you're having splashing in the puddles, and see your enthusiasm for life as you bound through the front door, they'll want to do it too. You'll get fitter, encourage each other and miss the rush hour. Pick different points to get out and you can easily measure your improvement. Make sure you build up to a run after you have been in the car, though. You could also do this if you get the bus home – jump out a few stops earlier than normal and walk home. Save on the bus fare, clear your head a bit and get some fresh air. Be careful, though – waiting at the bus stop in your go-faster running kit with price tags still on may earn you the nickname 'the nutter on the bus'.

Navy-style flight-deck circuit

This is the sort of all-round, full-body workout designed for a large group of fit sailors stuck at sea, with minimum space and equipment. You could do it with a couple of mates, or a sports team training in a cramped school hall in winter. You can pick any exercises but the following will work with only the participants' bodyweight required.

First exercise group:	Press-ups, crunchies and arm punching
Second group:	Star jumps, plank and lunges
Third group:	Half sits, knee press-ups, crunchies knee to elbow
Fourth group:	Bench dips, sit-ups and squats

Split the participants into groups of three and number them 1–3. All the number 1s in each group starts with press-ups. When they have completed the required amount (10–25 reps depending on fitness levels) they shout 'Change!' and move on to crunchies while number 2 starts press-ups. When number 1 has completed his crunchies, he shouts 'Change!' again and moves on to arm punching. Number 2 is doing crunchies and number 3 then joins in with press-ups. All three members work through the first exercise group two or three times depending on levels of fitness. Once that is done, take a breather for one minute and use the same principles to work through the second group of exercises.

It's like a domino effect – number 1 leads and takes charge and numbers 2 and 3 follow consecutively. Take it in turns to be number 1 so the same person is not leading all the time. It's a great workout for minimum space and equipment. If you have one person overseeing everyone, so much the better. They could time each exercise rather than relying on all the number 1s to shout 'Change!' If you want to exercise in a small or large group to create an atmosphere of hard work and get results, this is the one!

Dave's 'Simple but Special' – an easy way to start running

I've had unbelievable results with everyone who does this programme. It's so simple that first-time exercisers are a bit cynical. People seem to think only complicated routines work, but that's not the case.

A client came to me feeling unfit and sluggish. She wanted to get fitter, burn fat and improve her stamina. She wanted to be able to run but got out of breath after a few minutes so therefore got very despondent. We got together while she was on business in Bristol and managed about four training sessions. She needed a routine that could be done on her own while travelling around Europe. I explained the following routine to her and promised she would be running comfortably for 25 minutes without stopping. Within a short period she completed a 5-km run for charity, and was soon aiming to complete her first 10-km road race. Within a year she was in training for a half marathon.

This is a really simple but very effective way of improving your fitness levels and running abilities. It can also be very motivating if you just follow the simple routine, and as always be *consistent*. You can do this on a treadmill, on a sports field, in the park or simply around the streets. Make it last for 12–30 minutes depending on your levels of fitness. Just walk easy for one minute and then jog or walk hard for one minute. Do that continuously for your time chosen. For example, if you manage 20 minutes, that's 10 minutes walking and 10 minutes jogging alternately. Be careful, the first minute jogging might seem easy but as the session progresses it will be more of a challenge. You'll need to do it a few times to discover your pace judgement. You'll quickly improve if you manage two or three times a week. Three 20-minute sessions adds up to only one hour. You can rest for the other 167 hours left in the week!

The time will fly by with this routine. It's good because you have little targets to go for and it makes you focus on what you are doing. If you don't think you like running, or are a bit anxious but want to have a go, this will change your attitude. You'll see dramatic improvements if you stick to the guidelines and stay consistent.

As you feel more confident, stronger and your stamina improves you can make it a little more challenging. If your routine lasts for 20 or 30 minutes then don't change that, but try walking for a minute and jogging/fast walking for 1.5 minutes until your time is up. As you progress, keep the recovery to a minute but add on 30 seconds to the jog every week. Before you know it you'll be running for four minutes and walking for one over a period of 20 minutes. You can keep building in a progressive, measurable and satisfying way.

Club 100

This is a simple circuit consisting of 10 basic exercises, alternating between upper body, stomach/lower back and legs. All you do is work your way through each exercise and move on once you have completed 10 repetitions of each exercise. As always, spend a few minutes warming up and preparing, and likewise easing down on completion. Once you've done 10 reps on each of the 10 exercises then welcome to Club 100! Don't rush each exercise but try and give yourself a minimum amount of rest between each one. Time yourself the first time you do it, and try to improve your time as the weeks go on – only time it once every two or three weeks, though. If you want to make the workout a little more demanding then increase the reps on each exercise, or keep the reps to 10, but do it twice or three times as your stamina increases.

Press-ups	x10
Crunchies	x10
Squats	x10
Plank	10 seconds
Bench dips	x10
Sit-ups	x10
Step-ups	x10
Shoulder press	x10
Leg-raise plank	x10
Lunges	x10

Interval training

Interval training is bouts of intensive work with rests in between. The 'Simple but Special' on page 99 is a form of interval training related to running. You can work harder if you have planned rests between each bout of high intensity. You can do interval training with most aerobic workouts – try a 20-minute session of one minute easy and one minute hard on a bike, rower or treadmill. You could even do the same in the pool: swim a fast length followed by a slow length. Do that for 20 minutes and see how far you swim, or simply do 20 lengths alternating hard and easy. Try to achieve a higher intensity during the hard bout than you would during a single continuous bout of exercise. The recovery time should be long enough so the next hard interval can be done at the same speed as the previous one. Interval training should be done after your general fitness levels have been developed with longer continuous aerobic workouts.

This type of training can be done in short, intensive bursts and is very time-efficient. You could achieve as much in a 20-minute interval session as you could in a steady, continuous 40-minute workout! It will take a bit of self-discipline but will add variety to your regime, which is important.

The following is an example of interval training and could be done on your own or with a small group. Find your nearest football pitch and after warming up try the following: Decide how many laps of the pitch you are going to cover, anywhere between six and 10. Then find a challenging pace you can maintain lengthways and a very light jog widthways. If you decide to do 10 laps of the pitch, that works out at 20 fast runs and 20 easy jogs! Suck it and see the first time you do this and don't go off too fast. Try and find a pace that is a challenge but that you can maintain for the first through to the last hard interval run.

Group exercises

If you don't like to exercise alone and prefer a buddy, a small or large group for moral support then the following three examples are the answer. It takes self-discipline to exercise alone but it's more difficult to go home early if you're exercising with someone. You could still exercise alone twice a week, but once a week perhaps get together with some mates to add variety to your programme. I've used these three circuits in various ways for 25 years and they are perfect. They are simple, effective and fun, and can be adapted to suit anyone from beginners to experienced exercisers. You won't regret having a go!

Steady Eddies – exercise, run and rest

This works perfectly with a group of three, but it can be done on your own or with 30 participants or more! Give your participants numbers from 1 to 3. You can use the exercises from the Club 100 above, only this time number 1 starts off with a simple run out to a fixed point and back, taking 20–40 seconds. Meanwhile, number 2 carries out the first exercise, i.e. press-ups, while number 3 is resting. Therefore, the time on the exercise and rest is determined by the running time. When number 1 returns he/she replaces number 3 and rests, while number 3 takes over press-ups and number 2 moves from press-ups to running. After each exercise, run and rest, move on to the next exercise, i.e. crunchies.

Each participant works in the following order: rest, exercise and then run and back to rest in a simultaneous order. Each member will run 10 times, exercise 10 times and rest 10 times. Make sure you don't go off too fast; keep each run the same pace throughout, and the same tempo on all the exercises. If you only do a short run (say 20 seconds) that's fine, but remember – that means you'll only get a short rest! Make sure the person resting is encouraging the runner and exerciser to add some positive atmosphere.

This is a great circuit and really popular with any participants. It is easy to organise and is suitable for all levels of fitness. It's simple, it goes quickly, and is very effective for all-round fitness.

Crazy Gang – exercise and run

The same principles apply to this workout, but there are a few changes, i.e. there's no rest! It's more intensive and can be done with two or more people. The first participant runs while his/her partner exercises. When the runner gets back, simply swap over and continue to work your way through the exercises and runs. This is quite a challenge so make sure you have a few weeks of Steady Eddies under your belt. It will take a couple of goes to get a feel for your exercise tempo and pace judgement, but stick with it – it's simple, quick and effective.

Competitive circuit

This is a great workout for a large group, for a keep-fit class or even highly motivated athletes. It adds a bit of spice and competitiveness for the participants if they are that way inclined. It could also be used to measure improvement from the beginning to the end of pre-season training. The downside is that the participants may rush the exercises and good form could be lost in the enthusiasm. Any exercises can be used, but the Club 100 will work well.

Each group member carries out an exercise while one participant runs shuttles that last 30–40 seconds. Get the runner to collect small cones at various distances. Stop exercising when the runner has finished. The participants count up their number of reps and make a note, then move on to the next exercise until everyone has completed one run and all the exercises. The faster the runner runs, the less time his opponents have on each exercise, making them score less. Allow 20–40 seconds of rest between each stance. When all participants have completed the circuit and run, collect the scorecards and establish the positions. Every time I've experienced a group doing this circuit they always work extra hard and push themselves more than usual, or blatantly cheat on the numbers!

You can't beat exercising outdoors, and I recommend having a go before you make a big commitment to joining a gym or health club. Simple bodyweight exercises are functional and challenging, but they also provide a good foundation of fitness before you use any gym equipment. Bodyweight exercises will help improve your body awareness and tune in more to exercise. It may feel strange exercising at home – and it definitely requires more self-discipline and motivation – but the benefits outweigh the drawbacks by far. If you start exercising at home or outdoors and keep it up, you'll definitely be in a better frame of mind before you join a gym.

Chapter 16

Exercise routines for gym members

In this chapter you'll find plenty of exercise routines for those of you who have access to a gym or gym equipment. Don't start at the first one and try and work your way through them all. Read through all the routines, get a feel for a few and decide which is the most practical and enjoyable for you. If you find one you like then stick it out for 4–6 weeks – don't just randomly change between regimes. After a while, you'll discover the most practical and effective workout for you.

General fitness programme

Start with 15–25 minutes of continuous aerobic exercise, such as walking, rowing or cycling and maybe mix them up. Followed by:

Squats	2 x 15–20 reps
Bent-over row	2 x 15–20 reps
Chest press or press-ups	2 x 15–20 reps
Upright row	2 x 15–20 reps
Plank	2 x 15–20 seconds

Fat burn/general conditioning

This programme could take at least 40 minutes but could be adjusted by decreasing the time on bike, rower or treadmill. Try and work with the minimum amount of rest between each set of exercises. Warm up with 10 minutes on the bike, then:

Step-ups	3 x 15 reps

Press-ups	3 x 15 reps
Upright row	3 x 15 reps
10 minutes row	
Squats	3 x 15 reps
Chest press	3 x 15 reps
Bent-over row	3 x 15 reps
10 minutes treadmill	
Plank	3 x 15 reps
Hip raises	3 x 15 reps
Crunch and push	3 x 15 reps

Increased muscle tone

Squats	2 x 15–30 reps
Chest press	2 x 15–30 reps
Bent-over row	2 x 15–30 reps
Hip raises	2 x 15–30 reps
Press-ups	2 x 15–30 reps
Step-ups	2 x 15–30 reps
Upright row	2 x 15–30 reps

Strength-building

Squats	3 x 6–8 reps
Chest press	3 x 6–8 reps
Bent-over row	3 x 6–8 reps
Single leg hip raises	3 x 6–8 reps
Press-ups – with leg raise	3 x 6–8 reps
Shoulder press	3 x 6–8 reps
Upright row	3 x 6–8 reps
Crunch and push	3 x 6–8 reps

All-over workout

Spend five minutes on the bike to warm up, then run twice through the following routine before you move onto the row:

Step-ups	12 reps x2
Press-ups	12 reps x2

Bent-over row	12 reps x2
Squats	12 reps x2
Chest press	12 reps x2
Single arm bent-over row	12 reps x2
5 minutes row	
Crunch and push	12 reps x2
Planks	20–30 seconds x2
5 minutes treadmill	

Short and sweet

Spend five minutes on the bike, then:

Step-ups and bent-over row	2 x 20 reps
Chest press and crunchies	2 x 20 reps
5 minutes row	
Squats	2 x 20 reps
Press ups and hip raises	2 x 20 reps
5 minutes treadmill	
Upright row and planks	2 x 20 reps

Finish-line 5

5 minutes bike	Easy
5 minutes row	Hard
5 minutes walk/run	Easy
5 minutes bike	Hard
5 minutes row	Easy
5 minutes walk/run	Hard

The previous pages have given you ideas for a way ahead, but if you're still unsure, try the routines in the box overleaf.

In the third phase, each week should always consist of two strength workouts and two aerobic workouts. You can choose from finish-line 5, an interval session (see page 102) or any continuous aerobic exercise for the twice-weekly aerobic workouts, and mix them up.

The following routine will work well if you have had a break from exercise or are just starting out. It should last 15–22 weeks, and goes from home workouts to gym. It's planned in a progressive way to encourage

Phase	Fitness programme	Gym or home	Per week	Timeframe
Kick-start	Daily dose Club 100	Home	x5 x2 (optional)	4–6 weeks
First phase	General fitness programme	Either	x3	4–6 weeks
Second phase	Fat burn/ conditioning or increased muscle tone programme	Either	x3–4	3–4 weeks
Third phase	Strength training and either finish-line 5 or interval session or continuous aerobic exercise for 30 minutes	Gym	Strength x2 Finish-line 5/ Intervals x2	4–6 weeks

you to firstly woo exercise in, and build on endurance and general conditioning before moving on to strength work. Whatever your goals this is the perfect way to build a foundation for a life of exercise.

Don't expect the first programme you try to be perfect for you. It may take a bit of trial and error, but that's to be expected. As you gain in experience and fitness levels you'll find what works for you. Make sure you keep the main principles in mind: *safe*, *enjoyable* and *consistent* exercise is the key.

Two for the price of one exercises

The following exercises are additional to the 6FLs and are quite challenging, so don't try them until you have consistently improved your general strength and conditioning. They are a progression from the 6FLs and are classed as compound exercises, i.e. they work more than one major muscle group at a time. Don't feel you need to do these on top of what you're doing, but they are good if you're looking for more challenging exercises. They are a great way to raise the tempo of your workout and will certainly get your heart rate up. Versions of some of them have already been included in the earlier programmes.

The maximum amount of equipment you will need will be a weight training bar or dumbbells. It will be beneficial to buy adjustable ones so you can change the weight/resistance to suit you. These can be bought at any sports shop or fitness retailers. Make sure you purchase collars to ensure the weights don't slip off and cause injuries. To save money you could use old plastic drink containers filled with water to act as resistance. For the chest press you will need a sturdy bench.

Power clean

It sounds a bit extreme but you'll need to get comfortable with this exercise when you're using free weights to ensure you lift any weights safely. It develops legs, back, shoulders and arms.

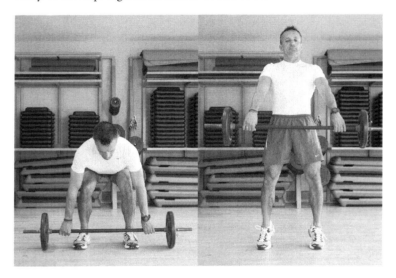

Start with your feet a shoulder-width apart and your heels down; squat down as if you are going to sit. Hold on to the bar/dumbbells or plastic containers with your knuckles up. Keep your back flat. Your shins should almost be touching the bar. Get your lower body engaged and feel like you are connected to the bar. Make sure your shoulders are loose, your arms are straight and look forward. Lift by straightening your legs, keeping your arms straight and the bar close to your body. When the bar is level with your chest drop your hips and bend your knees to lower your body. Rotate your hands and forearms under the bar and force the elbows forward and up. Rest the bar on your chest. To put the weight back down, first lower it to the thighs and use the same principles to lower to the floor.

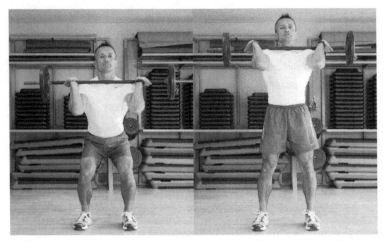

A variation on this is the deadlift, which works mainly the legs and lower back. The principles are the same as the power clean, but lift the weight to the hips only and lower to the floor.

Squat and shoulder press
This exercise works all your major muscle groups. It is very physically and aerobically demanding and will require a bit of co-ordination to

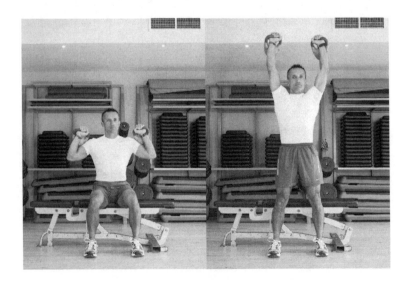

master. Your legs and shoulders are working simultaneously to push the weight above your head.

Stand with your feet a shoulder-width apart, holding the dumbbells just above your shoulders with your palms facing forward, your elbows in line and your wrists flat. Bend your knees into a squatting position until the back of your upper legs are parallel with the floor. Stand tall in one dynamic movement. As you do, extend your arms and raise the dumbbells above your head without locking your elbows. Lower the dumbbells slowly back level with your shoulders and repeat.

Single arm bent-over row

This is very similar to the bent-over row in the 6FLs, but it's done with one arm holding a dumbbell or weight and is a natural progression. It will work core muscles, mid back and the front of the arms.

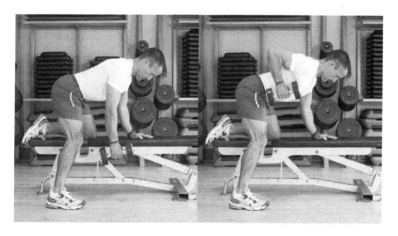

Place your left knee and left hand at right angles to your body on a bench and look down, right foot on the floor. Spread your bodyweight evenly. Lengthen your spine by pushing your bum away, stick your chest out and your shoulders down towards your hips. Very slightly bend your left elbow, think good posture and engage and tighten your stomach and lower back muscles. With your right hand naturally holding the weight underneath your right shoulder, bring the weight level with your chest. As you do, pinch your shoulder blades together and hold in that position for one second, then lower slowly. Don't use any momentum and don't let the shoulders rotate. Focus on the back muscles doing the work. Repeat and do the same on the opposite side.

Chest press or bench press

This exercise is similar to the press-up as it works the same muscle groups. A fabulous exercise for upper-body development; it can be done on a chest-press machine, with a barbell or dumbbells. Make sure you have someone to spot you and give you some support when you use free weights on this exercise.

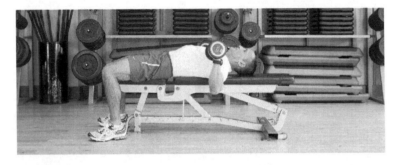

Lie on your back on the bench with your feet firmly on the floor and your knees bent at right angles. Hold the dumbbells with your knuckles up and your palms under the weight facing towards your feet. Keep both arms above your chest without the elbows locked. Lower the dumbbells slowly (4 seconds), and stop when the elbows are at 90 degrees. Make

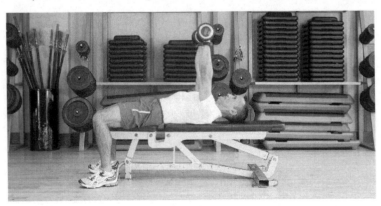

sure there is a definite stop (1 second) when your elbows are bent, then push the weight up in a more dynamic action (2 seconds). Repeat.

Progression and improving

I read a quote in a music book called *Effortless Mastery* by Kenny Werner. It says: 'It is good to view things as familiar or unfamiliar, rather than difficult or easy.' When you begin to exercise a lot of things may seem difficult (or unfamiliar) but it will get easier as you become more familiar with it. To progress you will need to make small changes and add challenges as your body adapts and becomes accustomed to your routine.

There is a training principle called 'progressive overload' used by athletes and professional sportspeople, which can be adapted for you. Exercise will slightly break your body down and build it back up if you have set the right challenges. Before focusing on improving your fitness levels, make sure you are exercising *consistently*. If you haven't exercised for a while then something as simple as walking will slightly improve your fitness levels. Going from no exercise or infrequent exercise to *consistently* exercising twice a week is classed as 'progressive overload' and will be enough to improve at first. Once you have wooed exercise into your life you'll have to add more challenges to your routine.

Age, health and general well-being will be deciding factors on how quickly your fitness levels progress, but staying *consistent* is the most important. There are four ways to add 'progressive overload' to your routine:

Frequency, intensity, time and type of exercise

Frequency

Simply exercising more will add intensity, if every week you do two sessions of walking/jogging and one of weights/resistance work, then just add another weight-training session every week. If you cycle to work twice a week, then add a cycle session at the weekend. Adding another bout of exercise during the week will force your body to make adaptations to your fitness levels and build your exercise awareness and confidence.

Intensity

Make your sessions more intensive by simply going from walking/jogging on the flat to adding some hills to your course, or simply move faster. If you are weight training have less rest between each exercise, maybe increase the repetitions or weight/resistance, or try adding some interval training to your aerobic work. Don't make the sessions last longer as well as being more intensive, though.

Time

Whatever type of exercise you are doing, keep the intensity the same but do it for longer. You could just add a few minutes on to your run, take a longer route on the bike, swim an extra five lengths or spend an extra 10 minutes at the gym.

Type

Changing the type of exercise can increase the intensity and overload but will take some thought. Going from weight machines to free weights is a good way, changing from squats to squats with weights is an example. Press-ups with your knees on the floor to hands and toes on the floor will make the exercise more demanding. You could simply do the same exercises but change the tempo. Try each exercise really slowly, and then after a few weeks do the same but increase the speed and tempo. If you are swimming then swim with a float between your legs or add a hill interval session to your running schedule.

The above principles will help you improve your fitness levels in a very effective way. Don't make the error of emptying your jar of enthusiasm and suddenly exercising more frequently, going for longer, running faster, lifting heavier weights with minimal rest all at once! Add the above ideas *one at a time*. If you are exercising twice a week, just change to three times a week until it's part of your routine, *then* increase the time exercising. After 4–6 weeks increase the intensity, and so on. This will ensure you progress and stay motivated.

Rest and relaxation

You might have spent some time being inactive and feel very keen to get started on your new exercise regime. However, rest and relaxation are an important part of your exercise plan. Following the guidelines in this book and wooing exercise into your life will naturally allow you to get enough rest between bouts of exercise. As you exercise more frequently and at a higher intensity you'll have to rest effectively to ensure you recover and improve.

If you are only exercising two or three times a week you should be getting enough rest to aid recovery. As you exercise more you'll get a better feel for what you are capable of and for how long. If you start to exercise for three or four times a week, make sure the sessions are spread evenly throughout the week. Rather than exercising every day from Monday to Thursday and then having three days off, exercise on Monday and Tuesday, rest on Wednesday, exercise Thursday and Friday, then rest on Saturday and Sunday. This will ensure you're exercising at your best.

The positive effects of exercise take place when you are resting. If you go from no exercise to exercising four days consecutively you risk overdoing it, getting injured or ill. Make sure you are wooing in the exercise and patiently building the intensity.

If you're exercising four days a week you'll inevitably exercise for two consecutive days. This is fine, but the trick is not to have two *hard* training days together. So, if you go for a hard run on a Monday don't try and mirror that session the next day. Either do a lighter and shorter run, or try light weights or resistance work. This will help you improve gradually and stop the boredom factor kicking in. When Wednesday comes around, have a total rest, eat healthily to encourage your body to recover. You'll be raring to go by Thursday!

Try the following workout:

Monday	Aerobic workout – cycling, walking, running or rowing
Tuesday	Resistance/strength training – 6FLs, weight training or bodyweight exercises
Wednesday	Rest or very light exercise
Thursday	As Monday
Friday	As Tuesday
Saturday	Rest or very light exercise
Sunday	Rest

This will ensure that the sessions are evenly spread out over the week and balanced with aerobic and strength work. Push the programme right by two days if mid-week exercise is not so easy and weekend exercise is more practical.

Wednesday	Aerobic workout
Thursday	Resistance/strength work
Friday	Rest or light exercise
Saturday	As Wednesday
Sunday	As Thursday
Monday	Rest or light exercise
Tuesday	Rest

If you are starting to woo exercise into your life you will naturally improve if you stay consistent. As your fitness levels improve you'll have to consider the points in this chapter in order to exercise effectively and help your body recover.

Chapter 17

What should I eat?

What you eat will play an important part in getting you healthy, active and fit. There's plenty of information about what to eat and what to avoid, and it's difficult to know where to start. As with exercise, we're going to work out what's best for you. A lot will depend on your eating habits since childhood and your relationship with food, as well as the eating habits of those close to you.

Forbidden foods
Keeping it simple and using a bit of common sense is a good start. It's easy to work out the food we should avoid but I'm always wary of telling clients what they shouldn't eat. If someone tells you that you can't eat chocolate or drink beer, you'll only spend your time thinking about how much you love chocolate and beer. So for now, just let it go and eat and drink what you want within sensible limits. We know what's good for us and what's bad, so let's focus on – yes, you guessed it – being *consistent*, and making some subtle changes.

Eat like a cow!
Next time you get the opportunity, watch how a cow eats. They spend all day munching away and slowly consuming their food. They take small mouthfuls, chew slowly, they love their fresh greens and don't think about anything else when they eat. They are in the moment! They never grab a quick bite, try to do other things at the same time, forget to eat and then consume large amounts to make up for it. Think about grazing like a cow when you eat – never go hungry, don't miss breakfast, eat smaller amounts and often, don't eat until you burst, eat slowly and

enjoy it. I know it won't always be practical – life gets in the way – so preparation is even more important. *Remember the 6Ps!*

Eating well is similar to exercising in terms of planning and organising your day. When food shopping, make sure you pick up some healthy snacks like fruit or nuts. When digging out your sports kit the night before, ensure you sort out those snacks for the next day or, better still, make your lunch for the following day. Not only is this cheaper, but you won't have to queue for your lunch and you could make a good healthy, enjoyable meal of your choice. It will take habit and self-discipline but it works. It's not about knowing what to eat, it's the planning that goes with it that's the real challenge.

How you're feeling will affect what you choose to eat. When you start exercising effectively and consistently you'll feel better about yourself. Eating good, healthy food will become easier. Don't suddenly try and stop eating your favourite chocolate or drinking real ale – it won't last! When you have a treat, savour it, enjoy the moment and reward yourself. Too much of one thing is never good for anyone.

'Drink water son, lions drink water!'

An old and bold Navy PTI told me a story from his childhood. He came from deep in the Welsh valleys and was as tough as old boots. He had run on numerous occasions for Portsmouth field gun crew and had a rugby ball permanently in his hands. His father was a Welsh miner and would take his young son to the labour club of an evening. As his father ordered a pint of Welsh bitter, his son would pull on his trouser leg and ask for a coke. The miner would pass his son a glass of tap water and say, 'Drink water, son. Lions drink water and you want to grow up big and strong don't you?'

The old miner had a point; if you are starting to exercise, then the chances are you need to consume more water. At least eight glasses a day is recommended to keep you hydrated. Don't wait until you're thirsty, keep a bottle of water close by and get into the habit.

'Perseverance is favourable.'

I Ching

Chapter 18

Exercise for life quiz

1. You are contemplating starting a new fitness campaign. Do you:

a) Decide to start next month, meanwhile as the date approaches gorge on chocolate until you promise you will stop forever.

b) Buy lots of magazines with celebrity get-fit-quick training tips, and book a beach holiday in two months to get you motivated.

c) Buy clothes too small for you, aim to get in them soon. Go out for a run. Thinking about it is no good, just get on with it.

d) Sit down, give yourself five minutes, think about what you want, and the effect it will have on your day-to-day routine.

2. You've decided to start your health and fitness campaign. Do you:

a) Rush out and buy gym membership for a year, hoping the cost will make you stick it out.

b) Buy new sports kit to get you started.

c) Find your old sports kit, go and try to do the same training session you did two years ago.

d) Sit down, ask yourself what you really want. Make small, subtle changes towards a healthy lifestyle and get into a positive frame of mind.

3. Your new fitness campaign is under way. Do you:

a) Exercise four or five times a week, for at least 40–50 minutes.

b) Religiously complete your celebrity 'get-fit-quick' three times a week, weigh yourself every day, cut out all treats, chocolate, cake and wine etc.

c) Exercise three times a week, make no change to your food and alcohol consumption as 'you've earned it'.

d) Arrange your days to make them slightly more active. Carry out three bouts of exercise per week that you find most enjoyable.

4. You are four weeks into your fitness regime. Do you:

a) Realise four times a week is too much, assume all healthy people are freaks and give up.

b) Note that you are feeling better, but it's taking longer than you think, therefore you decide to do less.

c) Decide that you are sticking with it, but that spare tyre hasn't gone yet, continue old eating and drinking habits.

d) Realise that the gradual process of a more healthy lifestyle is becoming easier. There are no visible changes but you realise that a 'slow but sure' process is the only way. You stay focused.

5. You are three months into your campaign. You have just returned from a two-week beach holiday. You had a break from exercise completely and have returned feeling all has gone to waste. Do you:

a) Give up completely feeling all your hard work has been wasted. Think about getting back to exercise three months before the next holiday.

b) Ignore the exercise programme, go back to your old ways, and start again in a couple of weeks. Because somehow it will be easier then!

c) Quickly get back in the gym, carry on where you left off before holiday, but train even harder to make up for feeling rubbish. Completely forget that you deserved a break and slip into the symptoms of a manic depressive.

d) Recognise that you made positive changes leading up to the holiday. Realise you have probably only lost about 10 per cent of your fitness levels. Ease back to your exercise programme, lowering the intensity until your previous fitness levels soon return.

6. You go to the gym three or four times a week. The majority of the time is spent running and walking on the treadmill, with a few half-hearted sit-ups to finish. You feel you are making no progress to your body shape. Do you:

a) Continue to do the same thing hoping there will be sudden results.

b) Look at using other equipment and classes, but keep on slipping back, feeling you have to go on the treadmill.

c) Add on some extra exercises after the treadmill work, and spend even more time in the gym.

d) Stop, reassess where you are. Talk to an advisor to review your progress. Spend less time on the treadmill and introduce resistance work to enhance your aerobic work.

7. You have been exercising consistently for six months with good results; it has become part of your routine. Your job has become more demanding, and you spend lots of time travelling. Do you:

a) Let the job take over your life, stop exercising and spend more time in work. Juggle work and exercise haphazardly, making infrequent visits to the gym, but trying to work harder to make up for lack of visits.

b) Decide to stop all exercise and start with more enthusiasm in a month.

c) Carry out a little bit of exercise in the week, but aim to train at the weekend when you could be with the family.

d) Make a plan at the beginning of the week for the most convenient times to exercise. Make small adjustments. Less time per workout, raise intensity. Take sports kit when away on business, exercise for 10 minutes in your hotel room. Stay consistent and persistent.

8. Exercise is a part of your life now. You have recently noticed a slight aching pain in the knee that causes discomfort and is worsening as you exercise. Do you:

a) Ignore it, continue to exercise hoping it will disappear.

b) Find other exercises that reduce the pain, continue but get frustrated and worry that you won't maintain your current fitness levels.

c) Take some time out from exercise, but don't seek advice.

d) Seek advice from your doctor or physiotherapist. Get treatment, work extra hard at your rehab, return to exercise programme with renewed enthusiasm.

If you've read this far you should be able to work out easily the best answers to all the questions!

Chapter 19

It's in the bag – you've nailed it!

Whether it's a physical, emotional, financial or spiritual goal, you can achieve whatever you want in life. It's as simple as that! It doesn't matter about your physical abilities, your background or past experiences – not one bit. It's down to you and your attitude. What do you want? Think positive, be positive and stay positive. Woo exercise into your life, start slowly, relish each challenge and keep moving forward.

Stay positive

You want to get fit, healthy and active and that will add nothing but positives to your life and the lives of those around you. It can completely change your attitude and enhance your life. You are not in competition with anyone or anything else. How will you fail?

It is down to you persevering and keeping your faith. As with all new challenges and goals there's always that last-minute big test to try your resolve! It's as if some unknown power is looking over you and asking 'Do you really want this? Can you do it?' Think about your final driving lesson before you passed your driving test… The finish line is always closer than you think. It seems a lifetime away when you're struggling and you think you will never get there. That's when many will turn away and walk off!

Don't ever give up. When you struggle make sure you smile at the hardship and challenges and accept them as part of the journey; there is no such thing as something for nothing. When you come out the other side you will be happy, rewarded and satisfied, and it will dawn on you what you are capable of.

It's only what you are entitled to.

Long-term possibilities, positives and advantages of being self-motivated to exercise on a regular basis:

- You feel good
- You'll be healthier and fitter
- It'll be easier to eat more healthily
- You'll savour treats and enjoy them more
- Your heart will be stronger
- You'll have a more effective immune system
- You'll be less prone to illness
- It will have a positive effect on the NHS!
- You'll recover more quickly from illness
- You'll feel more confident/attractive
- You'll sleep better
- You'll think more effectively
- You'll concentrate better
- You'll live and work more efficiently
- You'll make your Boss happy
- It may enhance your career…
- … and help you earn a better wage
- It will motivate/influence friends, family and work colleagues
- You'll relax more
- You'll enjoy a new interest
- It will boost self-belief
- You'll have more energy
- You'll have more stamina to keep up with your children
- It will influence your children to exercise
- You'll feel more alive and positive
- You'll be able to wear better clothes
- You'll achieve something you didn't think you could do
- You'll realise you can achieve whatever you want!

Long term negatives to being self motivated to exercise on a regular basis:

The End

Acknowledgements

I'd like to thank my Mum and Dad, Andy Roper, Sue O'Connell, Sonya Newland of Big Blu Books, Sam Lacey, Neil Harris, Mark Bolton Photography, Ibou Tall, all my clients, David Grant and everyone at Infinite Ideas Ltd, my daughters and of course my wife Jennie.

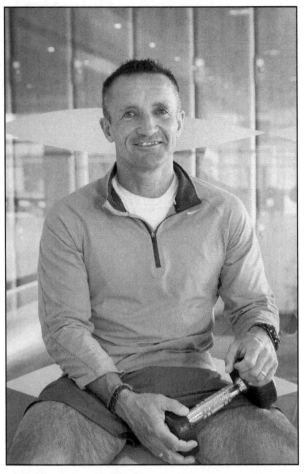

Dave Concannon spent 22 years in the Royal Navy serving as a fitness instructor at sea and ashore. He now runs his own fitness company in Bristol, providing motivation and guidance for anyone who wants to exercise. He is married with three daughters and a step daughter. In his spare time he likes to do nothing.

To contact Dave visit his website: **www.littledavefitness.co.uk.**